TITLE PAGE
The Metabolism Reset
Eat More, Burn More, Heal Your Body
How to Heal Your Hormones and Lose Weight Without Dieting

By Leonardo Lechuga

COPYRIGHT PAGE

DEDICATION

This book is dedicated to experience.

To the years studying health and nutrition simply because the human body fascinated me.

To the weights I lifted, the powerlifting I learned, and the lifestyle that shaped my youth.

To every athlete, every training partner, every coach, and every student who crossed my path—each with goals, dreams, challenges, and transformations of their own.

To the lessons absorbed in every gym, every mat, every struggle, and every breakthrough.

What I once thought was a "trick" for speeding up metabolism turned out to be a scientifically supported way of healing the body—from hormones to hunger signals to long-term health.

All of those years, all of those experiences, all of those people…

They led to this book.

Leonardo Lechuga spent decades studying health, nutrition, and human performance long before he ever considered writing a book. In his early years, he devoted himself to strength training, bodybuilding, and powerlifting—not for competition, but out of a genuine curiosity for how the human body works and how far disciplined training can push a person.

From age 21 into his mid-thirties, Leonardo immersed himself in fitness. When he entered the world of martial arts at age 39, everything expanded. Surrounded by elite fighters, dedicated athletes, and everyday people seeking weight loss, confidence, and transformation, he continued learning and teaching. As a martial arts coach, he helped students cut weight for competition, lose fat, rebuild their confidence, and reshape their lifestyles.

Over time, the patterns became undeniable.
The old dieting rules didn't work.
Starving didn't work.
Restricting didn't work.

But his whole-food, eat-every-two-hours approach did. Again and again.

What began as instincts from years of training and experimentation turned out to be strongly supported by metabolic and hormonal science. That discovery—and the desire to free people from diet propaganda—led Leonardo to write this book.

His mission is simple: to help people heal their metabolism, reclaim their health, and finally experience the freedom they were told was impossible.

TABLE OF CONTENTS

Explores how processed foods inflame, destabilize blood sugar, and damage hormones — and why whole foods heal.

How to read labels, avoid seed oils, choose clean ingredients, identify real olive oil, pick good salt, and avoid "healthy-looking junk."

PART IV — REAL RESULTS & A NEW LIFE

Chapter 26 — Success Stories & Real-Life Transformations

Composite stories showing how different types of people succeeded with this system.

Chapter 27 — Your New Life

A long-term plan for never dieting again and maintaining metabolic health for life.

INTRODUCTION

The Truth No One Told You About Losing Weight

Let me start with something bold:

If you've spent your whole life dieting, starving yourself, counting every calorie, and still ending up heavier, it's not your fault.

You were lied to.

For decades, the weight-loss industry has pushed one simple message:

"Eat less, move more."

And people believed it because it sounds logical. Simple. Clean. Except it fails — over and over — for nearly everyone who tries it.

Now, I'm not a scientist sitting in a lab coat writing theories. I'm someone who has lived a real life, been through real struggle, worked with real people, and helped real men and women change their bodies using a method that goes completely against what the diet world teaches.

And here's what I've seen:

When my students follow this system — eating whole foods every two hours — it works every single time. It doesn't matter if they're overweight, burned out, depressed, confused, or convinced their metabolism is "broken." The body responds the same way:

It wakes up. It burns more. It heals.

But you don't have to take my word for it.

The science backs this up too — strongly.

Studies from the National Institutes of Health show that within 72 hours of severe calorie restriction, the body begins metabolic adaptation (NIH, Dulloo & Jacquet, 1998). That's a fancy way of saying:

Your body slows down to survive.

It doesn't know you're trying to fit in a smaller pair of jeans
— it thinks you're starving to death. So it does what a good
survival machine does:

- Burns fewer calories
- Stores more fat
- Raises cravings
- Lowers energy
- Breaks down muscle

In fact, research published in the International Journal
of Obesity found that up to 80% of dieters regain all the
weight they lost within a year — and two-thirds regain more
than they originally lost.
That's not failure. That's biology.

So when people tell you, "Just eat less," I want you to
hear this clearly:
Starvation is not a weight-loss strategy. It's a weight-gain
strategy with a delay.

And here's where my personal experience comes in.
Over the years, I've had countless clients walk into my
program beaten down by every diet under the sun — keto,
fasting, low-carb, no-carb, points, shakes, detox teas, waist
trainers, you name it. They all showed up with the same
story:
"I lose weight for a little while… then it all comes back."
Some of them gained back 10, 20, even 40 pounds more.

But when I put them on a system that made absolutely
no sense to them at first —
Eat real food. Eat every two hours. No starvation. No
processed junk. No calorie counting.
— everything changed.

Not instantly.
The first two weeks are rough.

They feel full, uncomfortable, even irritated. They tell me, "I can't eat again already." Their hunger hormones are confused. Their stomach is deconditioned. Their metabolism is running like an engine that's been sitting in the cold too long.

But after that 10- to 14-day window, something incredible happens:

They show up hungry — right on schedule — every two hours.

Their cravings drop.

Their digestion improves.

Their energy increases.

Their mood stabilizes.

And the weight begins to fall off without suffering.

Why?

Because this method removes the single thing that destroys people's ability to lose weight:

inconsistency and scarcity.

When your body doesn't trust that food is coming, it hoards calories.

When it knows food is coming, it burns.

Harvard School of Public Health confirms this: whole foods increase the Thermic Effect of Food by up to 30% more than processed foods. Meaning your body literally burns more calories just digesting them (Harvard HSPH, TEF Overview, 2015).

Meal-timing research also shows that frequent eating stabilizes blood sugar and reduces insulin spikes (Journal of Nutrition, 2011), which means less fat storage and more stable energy.

The science says it.

My clients prove it.

And if you follow this book, you'll live it.

This isn't a diet.

This is a metabolic reset — a way to teach your body how to

burn fuel instead of storing it.

A way to break the cycle of losing and regaining weight.

A way to rebuild trust between you and your metabolism.

A way to eat more food and burn more fat — the way the body was designed.

And yes, you'll get tough love in this book.

Not because I want to be harsh, but because sugar-coating never saved anyone.

I'll tell you the truth the fitness industry won't:

Most diets fail before they even start because they're unsustainable and based on outdated science.

But this method works.

It's worked for every person I've ever trained who actually followed it.

And it'll work for you too — if you stick with it.

Now let's break the lies, rebuild your metabolism, and finally give you a system that works with your body instead of against it.

CHAPTER 1

THE DIET LIE EVERYONE BELIEVES

Let's get something straight right from the start:

Most people aren't struggling with weight because they're weak, lazy, or lack discipline.

They're struggling because they've been taught the wrong strategy for their entire lives.

The diet industry has convinced millions of people that the secret to weight loss is simple:

Eat less. Move more.

But here's the truth — and it's going to sting a little:

That advice is not only outdated, it's scientifically flawed.

And worse…it sets you up to fail before you even begin.

I've watched clients beat themselves up for years because they couldn't stick to starvation diets or extreme calorie cuts.

They thought THEY were the problem.

But the real problem is the lie they were sold.

THE CALORIE DEFICIT TRAP

Let's talk science for a minute.

Calorie-deficit dieting works in the short term — no one disputes that.

If you starve yourself, you'll lose weight at first.

But what most people don't know is this:

Your body adapts to that deficit FAST — and not in a good way.

According to research published in the journal Obesity Reviews, when calories drop too low, the body triggers something called adaptive thermogenesis — a survival mechanism that reduces the number of calories you burn at rest. (Rosenbaum & Leibel, 2010)

Leonardo Lechuga

Translation?

Your metabolism hits the brakes. Hard.

In fact, NIH studies found that metabolic rate can drop by 15–30% during aggressive dieting — and sometimes never fully recovers, even after normal eating resumes. (NIH, Dulloo & Jacquet, 1998)

So yes, eating less can make the scale move… but at the same time, it's teaching your body to become more efficient at storing fat and less efficient at burning it.

That's a losing game.

WHY STARVATION BACKFIRES EVERY TIME

Think of your metabolism like a fire.

If you throw fuel on it consistently, the flames stay strong. But if you stop feeding it?

It doesn't burn "hotter."

It dies down to preserve itself.

Your body works the same way.

It's engineered for survival.

When food becomes scarce:

- Your thyroid slows down
- Your hunger hormones go haywire
- Your cortisol (stress hormone) spikes
- Your body starts storing fat
- Your muscle tissue gets broken down for energy
- Your cravings intensify
- Your willpower collapses

This is biology — not willpower.

A landmark study from the Journal of Clinical Endocrinology & Metabolism showed that ghrelin (the hunger hormone) increases dramatically during calorie restriction, while leptin (the fullness hormone) plummets. (Klok et al., 2007)

Meaning?

You get hungrier.

You feel less satisfied.

Your body becomes obsessed with food.

And because cortisol is elevated, you store belly fat faster.

This is why people doing "1200-calorie diets" end up bingeing at night.

It's not a lack of discipline — it's the body's survival instinct.

THE REBOUND WEIGHT-GAIN PHENOMENON

Here's the part the diet industry really doesn't want you to understand:

Most people gain back MORE weight than they lost.

This is not anecdotal — the science is overwhelming.

The International Journal of Obesity reports that:

- 80% of dieters regain all weight lost within 12 months
- Two-thirds gain back more than they originally lost

Why?

Because once you come off a restrictive diet, your metabolism is slower than before.

But your appetite?

HIGHER than before.

Your body is trying to "catch up."

This is how people end up 20, 30, or 50 pounds heavier after dieting.

They didn't fail the diet.

The diet failed them.

Leonardo Lechuga

THE MENTAL DAMAGE DIETS CREATE

Let me talk to you as someone who's coached real people — not hypothetical lab subjects.

When clients come to me after years of dieting, they're:

- Mentally exhausted
- Afraid of food
- Confused about what's "allowed"
- Ashamed of their body
- Guilty after eating
- Stuck in an all-or-nothing mindset

The calorie-deficit lie trains people to fear eating.
To believe their body is the enemy.
To think weight loss requires misery.

And misery does NOT create consistency.
Consistency is the only thing that works.

There is nothing sustainable about weighing lettuce or starving before bed or fighting cravings all day.
No one lives like that long-term.

And if a system isn't sustainable?
It's not a solution — it's a setup.

WHY PEOPLE THINK THEY FAIL — AND WHY THEY'RE WRONG

I've had countless students say:
"I just don't have discipline."
"I lose motivation."
"I always fall off."
"I'm addicted to food."
"I have no self-control."

But what if I told you that almost every one of those statements is false?

It's not that they "lose motivation."
It's that their body was biologically incapable of sustaining the diet they were on.
It wasn't weakness.
It was biochemistry.

Imagine telling someone to hold their breath longer every day as a weight-loss strategy.
Sure, they can force it for a little while — but eventually the body will take over.

That's what starvation dieting is:
Holding your metabolic breath.

Eventually, the body will inhale — hard.

SO WHAT'S THE REAL PROBLEM?

Not the person.
Not their willpower.
Not their hunger.
Not their cravings.

The real problem is the strategy.
You cannot fight biology.
You cannot out-discipline your hormones.
You cannot starve your way to long-term success.
And you cannot expect short-term suffering to create lasting results.

If the method requires pain, restriction, and constant mental battles… it will fail.

Not because YOU failed — but because the method was never designed for humans in the first place.

Leonardo Lechuga

MY PERSONAL TAKE — AND WHY I WROTE THIS BOOK

I've used the Metabolism Reset Method with students and clients for years.

I didn't read it in a magazine.

I didn't pull it from a trend.

I didn't get it from the latest influencer pushing some detox tea.

I built this method by watching what works in real life.

I saw what happened when people stopped starving themselves and started feeding their body rhythm, real food, and consistency.

I saw energy return.

I saw cravings disappear.

I saw people lose weight eating more food than ever before.

I watched people go from:

"I'm always hungry"

to

"I'm hungry every two hours like clockwork."

That's not magic.

That's metabolism — finally working the way it was designed.

And once I saw what this method could do, I knew the truth needed to be written down, explained, and backed up with science so anyone could follow it.

This book isn't about dieting.

It's about breaking the cycle that has kept people stuck for years.

It's about giving your body what it needs instead of punishing it.

It's about using food as fuel — not fear.

It's about taking your power back.

CHAPTER 2

HOW THE BODY REALLY LOSES WEIGHT

Hormones, Hunger, Metabolism, and Why Everything You've Been Taught Was Backward

Before we go any further, I need to lay out the truth most people never learn:

Weight loss is not about calories — it's about hormones.

If you don't understand hormones, you will never understand metabolism.

And if you don't understand metabolism, you will spend your entire life dieting and gaining the weight back.

People think losing weight is a math problem.

In reality, it's a chemistry problem.

Now, I'm not going to drown you in textbook jargon.

I'm going to explain the biology in a way anyone can understand — and in a way that actually helps you change your life.

This chapter is where the "Eat More, Burn More" system stops sounding like a strange idea and starts sounding like common sense.

THE BODY'S REAL WEIGHT-CONTROL SYSTEM

Your body controls weight through a symphony of hormones.

They communicate constantly, and when they're balanced, weight loss becomes easy.

When they're disrupted, weight loss becomes almost impossible.

Here are the major players:

- Ghrelin — your hunger hormone
- Leptin — your fullness hormone
- Insulin — your blood sugar regulator
- Cortisol — your stress hormone

- Thyroid hormones (T3 & T4) — your metabolic thermostat
- Peptide YY & GLP-1 — your appetite suppressors
- Estrogen & Testosterone — body composition regulators

If these hormones aren't cooperating, you can eat "low calorie" all day long and lose nothing.

Conversely, if you balance them — especially using meal timing and whole foods — your body becomes a fat-burning machine.

Let's break them down one by one.

GHRELIN — THE HUNGER HORMONE THAT RESETS IN 14 DAYS

Ghrelin is the hormone that tells your brain:
"Hey, time to eat."

People with chaotic eating habits have chaotic ghrelin cycles.

People who skip breakfast don't feel hungry in the morning — not because they don't need food, but because ghrelin is dysregulated.

But here's the important part:
Ghrelin is highly trainable.

Clinical research published in Appetite (Cummings et al., 2004) shows that ghrelin follows a predictable rhythm based on your eating schedule.

This means:

- If you eat every 2 hours → ghrelin fires every 2 hours
- If you skip meals → ghrelin shuts down

- If you eat once a day → ghrelin fires once a day

When clients switch to the Metabolism Reset Method, their ghrelin system doesn't know what to do at first.

They feel overly full and uncomfortable.

But after 10–14 days?

Their hunger becomes predictable — the hunger that signals a healthy metabolism.

This is the "metabolic wake-up" you've seen in clients for years.

LEPTIN — THE FULLNESS SWITCH MOST DIETS DESTROY

Leptin is your fullness hormone — the hormone that tells you to stop eating.

When people are overweight or have been dieting for years, leptin becomes resistant.

Meaning:

- They never feel satisfied
- They overeat without meaning to
- They crave food even after meals

A study from The Journal of Clinical Endocrinology & Metabolism showed that calorie restriction lowers leptin drastically, which triggers:

- Slower metabolism
- More cravings
- Less satisfaction from food

THIS is why calorie-deficit diets backfire.

But here's the good news:

Whole foods + consistent eating patterns RESTORE leptin sensitivity.

Your body learns to recognize fullness again.

Leonardo Lechuga

Eating every 2 hours doesn't just "give your stomach a break" — it retrains your hormones to stop storing and start burning.

INSULIN — THE FAT-STORAGE SWITCH
Insulin decides whether your body:
A) stores fat
or
B) burns fat

Most people are stuck in "A" because they eat:
- High-sugar meals
- High-processed snacks
- Large meals too far apart
- Diets that spike blood sugar

Every big spike in insulin signals the body: "Store fat."

Frequent small meals of whole foods do the opposite. They keep insulin LOW and stable.

A study from the American Journal of Clinical Nutrition (Jenkins et al., 1989) found that eating smaller, more frequent meals significantly improved insulin response and reduced fat storage.

This means:

Your 2-hour system keeps insulin from spiking → which keeps fat from storing → which allows fat to burn.

It's not magic.
It's blood sugar control.

CORTISOL — THE HORMONE THAT MAKES YOU STORE BELLY FAT
Cortisol is your stress hormone.
And it LOVES storing fat — especially abdominal fat.

The Metabolism Reset

What raises cortisol?

- Starvation
- Skipping meals
- Over-exercising
- Stress
- Sleep deprivation
- Restrictive dieting

Research from the University of California (Epel et al., 2000) found that elevated cortisol increases cravings specifically for high fat, high sugar foods.

This is why starving yourself always ends in binge eating.

Eating consistent meals every 2 hours reduces cortisol levels because the body no longer believes it's in danger.

This alone improves fat loss dramatically.

THYROID HORMONES — YOUR METABOLIC ENGINE

The thyroid controls how fast your metabolism runs.

When you starve yourself:

- T3 drops
- T4 drops
- Metabolism slows
- Energy crashes
- Weight loss stops

And here's something most people don't know:

Your thyroid can take months to recover from even a short period of starvation dieting.

But eating predictable whole-food meals prevents that shutdown.

It signals the body:

"You are safe. You have fuel. No need to conserve."

This is why eating more (strategically) causes people to burn more.

THE THERMIC EFFECT OF FOOD (TEF) — THE SCIENCE BEHIND "EAT MORE, BURN MORE"

Whole foods require energy to digest, absorb, and convert into fuel.

This is called the Thermic Effect of Food (TEF).

Here's what science shows:

Food Type	Calories Burned During Digestion
Protein	20–30%
Whole carbs	5–10%
Processed carbs	0–3%
Fats	0–3%

Harvard School of Public Health found that whole foods cause double to triple the calorie burn compared to processed foods during digestion (Barr & Wright, 2010).

Meaning:

- Eating real food → metabolism increases
- Eating junk → metabolism slows

This is why your method works so well.
It uses natural biology to increase calorie burn — without starvation.

SO HOW DOES THE BODY REALLY LOSE WEIGHT?

Not by eating less.
Not by counting calories.
Not by starving.
Not by punishing yourself.

But by:

The Metabolism Reset

Balancing hormones
Stabilizing blood sugar
Lowering cortisol
Improving digestion
Increasing TEF
Keeping insulin stable
Training ghrelin cycles
Restoring leptin sensitivity
Feeding the body whole foods regularly
Creating metabolic trust

Weight loss isn't something you force.
It's something you ALLOW — by working with your biology, not against it.

COACH'S CORNER
Let me put this in plain talk.
Your body is not a calculator.
It's a living system.
And that system wants to survive — not be skinny.
If you treat your body like an enemy, it will fight back.
If you treat it like a partner, it will work with you.
Every time I've coached someone to eat real food consistently, their body responded EXACTLY the same way:

- More hunger
- More energy
- More fat burning
- Less craving
- Better sleep
- Better mood
- Better digestion
- Better metabolism

This chapter isn't theory.

It's the foundation of every success story you've ever seen in your program.

When you understand what your body wants, the weight comes off naturally — without suffering.

CHAPTER 3

HOW THE METABOLISM GETS DAMAGED

The Hidden Ways Dieting, Stress, and Daily Habits Slow Your Fat-Burning Engine

People don't wake up one day with a "slow metabolism." It doesn't just happen because of age or bad luck or "genetics." Metabolism gets damaged over time — slowly, quietly, and predictably.

And here's what most people get wrong:

You don't need to be overweight to have a broken metabolism. You can be tired, stressed, eating once a day, ignoring your hunger cues, and your metabolism can already be in the gutter without you realizing it.

In this chapter, I'm going to break down the real reasons metabolism slows down and why so many people end up stuck, frustrated, and gaining weight despite eating less food.

Once you see how metabolism gets damaged, you'll understand why our reset method fixes what nothing else can.

THE FIRST METABOLIC INSULT: SKIPPING MEALS

Let's start with the big one — the most common, the most destructive, and the one almost everyone has done:

Skipping meals.

Skipping breakfast, skipping lunch, getting "too busy" to eat — it all sends the same signal to the body:

"Food is unpredictable. Slow down."

The body, being built for survival, responds by lowering metabolic rate.

Science check:

Research from the American Journal of Clinical Nutrition (Farshchi et al., 2005) found that skipping meals leads to:

- Higher insulin levels

- Less stable blood sugar
- Increased hunger later
- Slower metabolic rate
- Greater fat storage

Meaning?

Skipping meals doesn't "save calories."

It trains the body to store calories.

I've seen this personally with clients over and over. People think they're being "disciplined" by skipping breakfast, when in reality they're basically hitting the brakes on their metabolism before their day even starts.

THE SECOND METABOLIC INSULT: PROCESSed FOOD

Let me be blunt:

The modern food industry is not your friend.

Processed foods:

- Spike insulin
- Cause cravings
- Slow digestion
- Destroy gut health
- Increase inflammation
- Lower thermic effect (you burn fewer calories eating them)
- Trick your hunger hormones

A study from the NIH (Hall et al., 2019) compared whole-food diets to ultra-processed diets and found that people eating processed foods automatically consumed 500 more calories per day without trying — and gained weight.

They weren't hungry.

They weren't bingeing.

They weren't emotional eating.

Their biology was reacting to the chemicals, additives, and hyper-palatable textures engineered into processed foods.

Your metabolism is designed for:

- Meats
- Vegetables
- Fruits
- Nuts
- Seeds
- Whole grains
- Real, natural foods

Not packaged snacks with 48 ingredients and a shelf life of three years.

THE THIRD METABOLIC INSULT: YO-YO DIETING

Yo-yo dieting — losing weight, gaining it back, trying again — is one of the WORST things you can do to your body.

Every cycle of restriction and regain damages metabolism further.

Science check:

A study in the International Journal of Obesity found that repeated cycles of dieting:

- Increase body fat percentage
- Reduce muscle mass
- Increase cortisol
- Disrupt hunger hormones
- Slow metabolic rate
- Make future weight loss harder

Think about what that means:

Every time you diet and fail, weight loss becomes harder the next time — not because you're weaker, but because your biology has adapted.

This is why people say:

"I used to lose weight easily when I was young… now nothing works."

It's not age.

It's accumulated metabolic stress.

THE FOURTH METABOLIC INSULT: CHRONIC STRESS

Stress is not just a feeling.

It's a hormonal state — one dominated by cortisol.

Cortisol tells the body to:

- Store belly fat
- Hold onto energy
- Increase cravings
- Reduce muscle-building
- Disrupt sleep
- Slow digestion

A study from UC San Francisco (Epel et al., 2000) showed that people with high cortisol are significantly more likely to gain abdominal fat — even if they don't eat more.

Let me repeat that:

Stress alone can make you gain fat.

Now combine stress with:

- skipping meals
- poor sleep
- processed foods
- restrictive dieting
- long work hours
- family responsibilities

This is a metabolic disaster.

The Metabolism Reset

Your body wasn't built for 2025-level stress.
It reacts the same way it did 10,000 years ago — by preparing for famine and danger.

THE FIFTH METABOLIC INSULT: SLEEP DEPRIVATION

Sleep is when:

- Hormones reset
- Hunger signals balance
- Stress levels drop
- Muscles repair
- Fat is mobilized
- Metabolism restores

Without enough sleep, the following happens:

- Ghrelin increases → you get hungrier
- Leptin decreases → you don't feel full
- Cortisol rises → you store fat
- Insulin sensitivity drops → you store even more fat

A 2010 study in the Annals of Internal Medicine found that people who sleep less than 6 hours burn 55% less fat while dieting.

Meaning:
You could be eating the same amount, doing the same things, and still lose half the fat simply because you're tired.

That's how powerful sleep is.

THE SIXTH METABOLIC INSULT: EATING TOO LITTLE FOR TOO LONG

This is the one most people NEVER expect.

Leonardo Lechuga

Eating too few calories for too long crushes your metabolism.

Your body thinks there's a famine, so it:

- Reduces metabolic rate
- Protects fat
- Burns muscle
- Lowers thyroid hormones
- Boosts hunger
- Slows digestion

This is not theory — this was proven in the famous Minnesota Starvation Study (Keys et al., 1950), where healthy men put on extreme calorie restriction experienced:

- Depression
- Weakness
- Obsession with food
- Metabolic slowdown
- Hormonal imbalance
- Fat retention
- Rebound weight gain

This is EXACTLY what modern dieters experience.

And the worst part?

Some never recover their full metabolic rate.

That's the punishment for starving your body:

You gain weight easier for the rest of your life…
until you fix the damage.

THE SEVENTH METABOLIC INSULT:
INCONSISTENT EATING HABITS

One day you eat breakfast.
One day you don't.
One day you eat at 11 p.m.
One day you eat nothing until 4 p.m.

The Metabolism Reset

One day you snack all day.
One day you don't.
One day you're on a diet.
One day you're "taking a break."
This inconsistency is brutal on the metabolism.
The hunger hormone ghrelin becomes unstable.
Insulin spikes randomly.
The thyroid gets confused.
Cortisol rises.
Blood sugar yo-yos.
The digestive system becomes irregular.
Your body wants predictability.
It wants rhythm.
It wants routine.
This is why your 2-hour system works so beautifully — it gives the body the stability it has been starved for (no pun intended).

THE EIGHTH METABOLIC INSULT: LACK OF MUSCLE

Muscle is metabolically active tissue.
The more muscle you have, the more calories you burn at rest — even while doing nothing.
When you starve yourself, you lose muscle.
When you do tons of cardio without eating enough, you lose muscle.
When you get older and inactive, you lose muscle.
Less muscle → slower metabolism → easier fat gain.
A study in the American Journal of Physiology found that every pound of muscle burns roughly 6–10 more calories per day at rest.

That may not sound like much, but over 20–30 pounds of muscle, it adds up fast.

This is why people who lose weight through starvation often gain it back — but as fat, not muscle.

THE COMPOUND EFFECT OF DAMAGE

Now imagine someone who:
- Skips breakfast
- Eats processed foods
- Has a history of dieting
- Works long stressful hours
- Sleeps poorly
- Eats inconsistently
- Doesn't exercise
- Has lost muscle
- Lives in chronic cortisol

That person is not "bad at dieting."

Their metabolism is shut down because life has been beating it up for years.

And THIS is the person who benefits most from the Metabolism Reset Method.

Not because it's magic,

but because it addresses almost EVERY cause of metabolic damage…

at the same time.

COACH'S CORNER

Most people are not overweight because they "eat too much."

Most people are overweight because:
- They're stressed
- They're sleep-deprived

- They skip meals
- They're eating the wrong types of food
- They've dieted too many times
- Their hormones are wrecked
- Their metabolism is confused
- Their body is scared to burn energy

I've never met a single person who had a slow metabolism "for no reason."

Every person had a story — a life — that explained exactly how they got there.

This chapter is not about blame.

It's about understanding.

You cannot fix what you don't understand.

But once you see the damage clearly, you can reverse it.

And that's where the next chapter comes in — it explains WHY your 2-hour whole-food system heals all of this.

CHAPTER 4

WHY EATING EVERY 2 HOURS WORKS

The Metabolic Logic Behind "Eat More, Burn More"

Most people's first reaction to the Metabolism Reset Method is pure disbelief.

"Eat every two hours? Isn't that too much?"

"Won't I gain weight?"

"How does eating more help me burn fat?"

I've heard all of it. Every objection. Every fear. Every misconception.

And I get it — because the entire world has been conditioned to think less food = more weight loss.

But the truth is the opposite:

More of the RIGHT food, eaten at the RIGHT time, creates a metabolism that burns fat instead of storing it.

This isn't a gimmick.

This isn't a fad diet.

This isn't a trick.

It's how the human body is biologically designed to function.

In this chapter, I'm going to break down the science, the logic, and the real-world results behind this method.

When you understand why it works, you'll never let yourself fall back into starvation or crash dieting again.

THE PRINCIPLE OF METABOLIC TRUST

Let's start with the foundation — the concept everything else rests on:

The body burns more when it trusts that food is coming.

If your body thinks you're in danger of not eating, it slows down every system involved in energy use.

The Metabolism Reset

It prepares for famine.

It preserves fat.

It reduces metabolism.

It increases fat storage.

It protects energy at all costs.

Your body has one mission:

Keep you alive.

It doesn't care about your goals.

It doesn't care about your summer plans.

It doesn't care about your jeans.

So when you skip meals or go hours without eating, the body interprets that as a survival threat.

But when you feed it consistently — every 2 hours — everything changes.

The body says:

"Food is abundant. I'm safe. I can burn freely."

This is what I call metabolic trust.

It is the single most important factor in sustainable fat loss.

THE SCIENCE OF MEAL FREQUENCY AND BLOOD SUGAR STABILITY

Every time you eat, your blood sugar rises slightly.

When you go too long without eating, blood sugar crashes.

These swings cause:

- Hunger
- Cravings
- Insulin spikes
- Fat storage
- Energy crashes
- Mood changes

A study published in the Journal of Nutrition (2011) found that eating smaller, more frequent meals:

stabilizes blood sugar
improves insulin sensitivity
reduces hunger
reduces overeating
increases metabolic output

Your body LOVES stability.

Predictable eating = predictable hormones = predictable fat burning.

When you eat every 2 hours, your blood sugar stays balanced.

This keeps insulin — the fat-storage hormone — low and steady.

Low insulin = fat burning.

High insulin = fat storage.

It really is that simple.

WHY SMALL, FREQUENT MEALS SPEED UP DIGESTION

People think eating every 2 hours "overloads the stomach."

Nope.

What actually happens is this:

Your digestive system becomes more efficient.

- Enzymes activate faster
- Stomach emptying improves
- Gut motility increases
- Nutrient absorption becomes smoother
- Bloating decreases
- Metabolism accelerates

This is why clients who first say:

"I'm too full to eat again."

Later say:

"I'm starving right on schedule at two hours."

Their digestive system learns the rhythm.

It adapts.

It speeds up.

This is metabolic training in action.

And research backs this up:

A study in the American Journal of Gastroenterology showed that structured meal timing improves GI function and increases the rate of gastric emptying (Monnikes et al., 2001).

Translation:

Eating more often makes the body better at processing food.

WHY THE FIRST TWO WEEKS FEEL HARD

Let me explain the "misery phase" you've seen hundreds of times.

When someone starts the 2-hour eating plan:

- Their stomach is deconditioned
- Their hunger hormones are chaotic
- Their metabolism is slow
- Ghrelin isn't firing on schedule
- Insulin is unstable
- Digestive enzymes are weak
- Cortisol is elevated
- Leptin is confused

They are not broken — they are untrained.

The first two weeks feel uncomfortable because the body is waking back up.

Here's what's happening physiologically:

Ghrelin begins to establish rhythm

Leptin begins to send correct signals

Digestive enzymes increase

Insulin stabilizes

Cortisol drops
Thermic effect increases
Thyroid function improves
Metabolism shifts from storage to burn mode
This is the metabolic equivalent of:
"Hold on… recalibrating…"
Once the recalibration is complete — hunger appears on schedule, energy improves, and fat loss accelerates.

THE THERMIC EFFECT OF WHOLE FOODS

Whole foods burn calories just by being digested.
Let's repeat the TEF chart for emphasis:

Food Type	Calories Burned Digesting
Protein	20–30%
Whole carbs	5–10%
Processed carbs	0–3%
Fats	0–3%

Your method emphasizes:
- lean proteins
- whole fruits
- vegetables
- nuts
- seeds
- natural carbs
- simple whole-food snacks

This means the body is burning calories:
- all day
- every meal
- every snack
- every time digestion activates

The Metabolism Reset

A 2010 study from Harvard confirmed that whole foods increase metabolic rate significantly more than processed foods (Barr & Wright, 2010).

This is why people eating your plan often say:

"I feel like my body is burning all the time."

It is.

HOW THE 2-HOUR SYSTEM FIXES HORMONAL DAMAGE

Let's break down each hormone again and explain EXACTLY how the method heals them.

Ghrelin (Hunger Hormone)

Eating every 2 hours retrains ghrelin to fire consistently. This creates stable appetite, predictable hunger, and reduces overeating.

Leptin (Fullness Hormone)

Whole foods + predictable eating restore leptin sensitivity. People feel satisfied again — not craving nonstop.

Insulin (Blood Sugar Hormone)

Smaller meals prevent spikes.

Whole foods prevent surges.

Stable insulin = fat burning mode activated.

Cortisol (Stress Hormone)

Consistency signals safety.

Safety lowers cortisol.

Lower cortisol = belly fat reduction + hormonal balance.

Thyroid (Metabolic Hormones)

Leonardo Lechuga

Regular nutrition prevents thyroid slowdown and improves T3/T4 production.

GLP-1 & Peptide YY (Satiety Hormones)
These increase with whole foods and frequent eating — the same hormones drugs like Ozempic artificially stimulate.
Your method accomplishes the same effect naturally.

WHY EATING MORE LEADS TO BURNING MORE
Here's the shortest, realest explanation:
When the body receives:
- consistent fuel
- predictable timing
- real food
- balanced macros

… it stops acting like a creature trying to survive starvation
and starts acting like a machine built to perform.
Starvation creates:
- slow metabolism
- cravings
- mood swings
- fat storage
- muscle loss
- rebound weight gain

Eating frequently creates:
- faster metabolism
- stable energy
- natural hunger
- better digestion
- fewer cravings

- fat mobilization

This isn't theory.

This is what you've witnessed in every client who actually followed the program.

THE REAL REASON THIS METHOD ALWAYS WORKS

Because it addresses EVERY factor that controls metabolism:

Hormones

Digestion

Blood sugar

Cortisol

Thyroid

Muscle preservation

Hunger signals

Satiety signals

Thermic effect

Consistency

Metabolic trust

And unlike every crash diet on earth, this method is:

- sustainable
- realistic
- enjoyable
- science-based
- predictable
- psychologically healthy
- physiologically sound
- metabolically restorative

This is not a "diet."

This is a retraining protocol for your metabolism.

And once the metabolism is trained correctly…

the weight comes off without force.

COACH'S CORNER

Let me speak as your coach for a second, not your scientist.

I've seen people go from exhausted, stressed-out, craving junk, skipping meals, and eating once a day…

to energized, confident, hungry on schedule, burning fat, and feeling GOOD for the first time in years.

All from eating whole foods every two hours.

The hardest part is getting them to trust the process. The body is ready long before the mind is.

Once they get past the mental block — once they stop fighting their biology — once they start feeding the machine instead of starving it…

it's over.

The weight doesn't stand a chance.

This method works because it's based on how the human body is meant to function — not how the diet industry wants you to suffer.

CHAPTER 5

THE 2-WEEK TRANSITION: FROM MISERABLE TO METABOLICALLY ALIVE

Why the Beginning Feels Like Hell — and Why That's the Best Sign You're Finally Healing

If you've ever started the Metabolism Reset Method — or watched one of my clients begin it — you already know something weird happens in the first couple of weeks.

It goes like this:

Week 1:

"I'm so full. Why are you making me eat again?"

Week 2:

"I still feel stuffed… but I'm starting to notice I'm hungry right before my next meal."

After Day 10–14:

"I don't know what happened, but now I'm starving every two hours."

This shift isn't random.

It's not psychological.

And it's definitely not a coincidence.

What you're witnessing is the metabolism rebooting itself — turning back on after years of being slowed down, suppressed, confused, or damaged.

This is the moment the body stops surviving and starts performing.

Let's break it down.

WHY WEEK ONE FEELS MISERABLE

People expect a new meal plan to feel exciting, motivating, energizing.

But that's not what happens in Week 1.

Week 1 feels like punishment.

And here's the truth most coaches won't tell you:

Week 1 is SUPPOSED to feel uncomfortable.

If it doesn't, you weren't broken enough to need the reset in the first place.

There are several reasons for the misery — and every single one is biological.

1. THE STOMACH IS DECONDITIONED

Most people who come into this program have spent YEARS:

- skipping breakfast
- eating one big meal at night
- grazing on snacks instead of meals
- bingeing after long gaps
- eating inconsistently

Their stomach is not used to receiving food every 2 hours.

When you suddenly begin feeding it real whole foods at regular intervals, the stomach responds like any muscle that's been neglected:

"What the hell is this?"

It stretches.

It activates.

It produces enzymes again.

It wakes up.

That "too full" sensation isn't overeating — it's reactivation.

A 2002 study from Gut (Jones et al.) found that people who chronically under-eat have slower gastric emptying — meaning food sits in their stomach longer.

Week 1 is the stomach retraining itself.

2. GHRELIN IS NOT FIRING CORRECTLY

Remember ghrelin?

The hunger hormone that runs on a schedule?

Well, most people's ghrelin rhythm is destroyed.

If they're used to eating once or twice a day, ghrelin fires:

- at the wrong times
- too strongly
- or not at all

So when you ask them to eat every 2 hours, ghrelin isn't ready.

It's confused.

A 2004 study published in Appetite showed that ghrelin quickly adjusts to eating schedules — but it takes roughly 10–14 days to fully synchronize.

During those first 10 days:

- They're not hungry when it's time to eat
- Then suddenly they're starving at random times
- Hunger cues feel unreliable
- Fullness feels exaggerated

This is the SIGN of ghrelin rebooting.

3. LEPTIN IS NUMB OR RESISTANT

Leptin — the fullness hormone — gets damaged from:

- starving
- yo-yo dieting
- eating junk food
- chronic stress
- poor sleep

So in Week 1, leptin is basically unreliable.

It either:

- tells you you're full too early
- doesn't tell you you're full at all

- or flips between the two

Whole foods + consistent eating begin to restore leptin sensitivity, but it takes time.

Week 1 is the recalibration period.

4. THE METABOLISM IS STILL IN "SURVIVAL MODE"

You can't starve your body for years and expect it to immediately start burning fuel efficiently.

When people start this method, metabolism is usually:

- cautious
- suppressed
- energy-conserving
- in a defensive state

Week 1 is the body watching and waiting:

"Are we actually going to keep getting real food? Or is this another famine disguised as a diet?"

It's like an abused dog flinching even when you're trying to feed it.

Once your metabolism realizes you're actually providing consistent nourishment, it begins to change — FAST.

5. DIGESTION IS WAKING UP

People think their digestive system is "slow."
It's not slow — it's underused.

When you begin eating every 2 hours:

- gastric emptying increases
- enzymes activate
- gut motility improves
- the microbiome begins shifting
- inflammation lowers

These changes can feel like:

- fullness
- bloating
- heaviness
- sluggishness

This is NORMAL.

It's the system warming up.

THE TURNING POINT: DAY 10 TO DAY 14

Something happens between Day 10 and Day 14 that shocks people every single time:

Their hunger returns — like clockwork, every 2 hours.

This is the moment the metabolism transitions from "survival mode" to "performance mode."

Let's break down what's happening.

1. GHRELIN RESETS

Your hunger hormone finally syncs with your eating pattern. Suddenly:

- Hunger becomes predictable
- The stomach empties on time
- The body begs for food right at the 2-hour mark

The body moves from reactive hunger → rhythmic hunger.

This is one of the biggest signs of metabolic health.

2. DIGESTION SPEEDS UP

Clients who once complained about being "stuffed" now say:

"I can't believe I'm hungry again."

"I actually feel empty at the 2-hour mark."

"I'm craving whole foods."

Digestive enzymes are firing.
Stomach emptying is efficient.
Nutrient absorption is improved.
Inflammation is reduced.

The GI system is now trained.

3. INSULIN IS STABILIZED

Blood sugar is no longer swinging wildly.
This means:

- no more crashes
- no more emergency cravings
- no more binge urges
- no more nighttime hunger

This stability is what allows fat-burning to begin happening around the clock.

4. CORTISOL DROPS

The body stops panicking.
It stops holding fat.
It stops sending stress signals.
It stops conserving energy.

When cortisol drops, metabolism rises.

5. THE "BURN SIGNAL" ACTIVATES

Once the body trusts:

- food is coming
- meals are predictable
- there's no famine
- hormones are regulated
- digestion is efficient

… it unlocks something powerful:
Fat mobilization.

The Metabolism Reset

This is when the scale begins to move.

When clothes fit differently.

When clients feel lighter.

When energy improves dramatically.

This is the "alive" feeling clients talk about.

THE PSYCHOLOGICAL SHIFT

Around two weeks in, something changes in people's MINDS too.

They stop fearing food.

They stop feeling guilty about eating.

They stop thinking in calories.

They stop worrying about "falling off."

Because now they FEEL the difference.

And once someone FEELS their metabolism working…

they never want to go back to starvation again.

WEEK-BY-WEEK BREAKDOWN

Here's exactly what most people experience:

WEEK 1

- Fullness
- Discomfort
- Confusion
- Stomach resistance
- Hormonal chaos
- Low motivation
- Doubt
- Fatigue
- Mental resistance ("This can't be right…")

This is normal.

This is the detox from diet culture and metabolic dysfunction.

WEEK 2
- Less fullness
- Sudden hunger patterns emerging
- Improved digestion
- Stabilized mood
- More energy
- Fewer cravings
- Better sleep
- More predictable appetite

The body is adapting.

DAY 10–14: THE METABOLIC TURNING POINT
- Hunger every 2 hours
- Efficient digestion
- Stable energy
- Clearer thinking
- Less bloating
- Better bathroom habits
- Improved mood
- Reduced cravings
- Beginning signs of fat loss

This is when everything "clicks."

COACH'S CORNER

If you quit in Week 1, you will never experience what your body is truly capable of.

You have to push through the discomfort.

You have to trust the system.

You have to let your body relearn what it forgot.

The Metabolism Reset

Every person I've trained who stuck with this method —
every single one — got the same result:

Hunger returned.

Energy increased.

Fat started burning.

Life got easier.

And once the body wakes up, it does NOT want to go back
to sleep.

This is the price of becoming metabolically alive:

→ You have to get uncomfortable before you get
unstoppable.

But once you hit that transition point, the rest of this
journey becomes a whole different game.

CHAPTER 6

WHY STARVATION FAILS EVERY TIME

How Eating Less Destroys Metabolism, Increases Fat Storage, and Guarantees Weight Regain

If there is one chapter in this entire book I want you to read twice, it's this one.

Because THIS is where most people destroy themselves without realizing it.

Every time someone says:

"I'm just going to eat less."

"I'll fix my diet starting Monday."

"I'm cutting calories down to 1200."

"I need to starve myself for a bit to reset."

… they are setting themselves up for failure.

Not because they lack discipline, but because biology will always beat willpower.

You cannot outsmart the human survival system.

You cannot bully your metabolism into submission.

You cannot starve your way into long-term weight loss.

Your body is older, smarter, and more stubborn than any diet plan — and the moment you take food away, it activates systems designed to keep you alive at all costs.

And those systems do NOT care about your weight-loss goals.

THE STARVATION RESPONSE: BUILT-IN FAILURE FOR DIETS

Let's go all the way back to evolution.

Humans weren't built for "three meals a day" or Uber Eats or drive-thru windows.

They were built for scarcity — for long periods without food.

The Metabolism Reset

So when food disappears, the body says:

"We're in danger. Slow everything down."

This reaction is called metabolic adaptation, and it begins shockingly fast.

A major study by the National Institutes of Health (Dulloo & Jacquet, 1998) found that when calorie intake drops too low:

- Metabolic rate decreases
- Fat burning slows
- Hunger increases
- Energy declines
- Hormones go out of balance
- Fat storage increases

It's the body's way of protecting you.

This means:

The more you starve, the LESS you burn.

The more you restrict, the faster your metabolism shuts down.

Starvation doesn't create weight loss —

it creates metabolic panic.

WHY THE SCALE DROPS FAST AT FIRST — AND WHY THAT'S A TRAP

Most people fall for the oldest trick starvation pulls:

rapid early weight loss.

This happens because:

- Your body dumps water
- Your glycogen stores empty
- You burn muscle tissue
- You lose sodium

None of this is fat loss.

In fact, the first 5–10 pounds are almost ALWAYS water and muscle — the two things you need to KEEP to support a fast metabolism.

Leonardo Lechuga

A 2010 study in Annals of Internal Medicine found that calorie-restricted dieters lost significantly more lean muscle mass than fat during the first two weeks.

So yes — the scale drops.

But here's the real truth:

 Fast weight loss = slow metabolism.

It is a trap.

A psychological hook.

A temporary illusion.

And as soon as you return to normal eating?

Your body rebounds — hard.

CORTISOL: THE HORMONE THAT MAKES YOU GAIN BELLY FAT

When you starve yourself, your body produces more cortisol — your stress hormone.

Elevated cortisol causes:

- Increased fat storage
- Especially in the belly
- Muscle breakdown
- Insulin spikes
- Sugar cravings
- Mood swings
- Water retention
- Slower metabolism

Research from UCSF (Epel et al., 2000) showed that high cortisol levels directly correlate with abdominal fat gain — even if calorie intake is low.

Read that again:

Even if you're eating less, cortisol can make you store MORE.

Meaning:

Starvation = belly fat

Stress = belly fat

Dieting = belly fat

You cannot burn fat while producing high cortisol. Period.

STARVATION DESTROYS MUSCLE — AND MUSCLE IS YOUR METABOLIC ENGINE

When the body senses starvation, it doesn't burn fat first.

It burns MUSCLE.

Why?

Because:

- Fat = long-term energy storage
- Muscle = expensive tissue

Muscle burns calories even while resting, so your body sees muscle as a liability during famine.

A study in the American Journal of Clinical Nutrition confirmed that up to 45% of weight lost on calorie-restricted diets comes from lean muscle tissue.

And here's the brutal truth:

Less muscle = slower metabolism

Slower metabolism = easier fat gain

Easier fat gain = rebound weight

It's a mathematical certainty.

When you starve yourself, you lose the very thing that burns calories.

THE THYROID SHUTDOWN

Your thyroid controls metabolic speed.

During starvation:

- T3 drops
- T4 drops
- Thyroid conversion slows

- Metabolic rate plummets

This effect is so strong that even brief periods of starvation can suppress thyroid output for months.

A study in Metabolism (1990) showed that thyroid hormones decrease within DAYS of calorie restriction.

This is why people feel:

- cold
- fatigued
- depressed
- mentally foggy
- unmotivated
- stuck

This isn't lack of discipline —
it's your thyroid slowing everything down to keep you alive.

THE GUT SHUTS DOWN TOO

People think constipation or bloating during dieting is because they're "eating less."

No.

It's because:

- digestion slows
- stomach emptying slows
- gut motility decreases
- microbiome diversity drops

A 2011 review in Nutrients found that low-calorie diets alter the gut microbiome in ways that make fat storage MORE efficient.

Meaning:

Starvation teaches your body to STORE more from LESS food.

That's the opposite of weight loss.

The Metabolism Reset

THE BRAIN'S RESPONSE: OBSESSION & CRAVINGS

When food intake drops too low, your brain goes into survival mode:

- You obsess over food
- You think about cravings nonstop
- Willpower collapses
- Your reward centers activate
- High-calorie foods become almost irresistible

This is a neurological reaction driven by dopamine and serotonin changes — NOT weakness.

A 2016 study in Cell Metabolism (Rosenbaum et al.) found that dieting increases brain sensitivity to food cues.

This means:

Your brain becomes MORE obsessed with food the LESS you eat.

This is why "1200 calorie people" always binge at night.

It's not lack of discipline — it's biology screaming for survival.

THE REBOUND EFFECT: WHY PEOPLE GAIN MORE THAN THEY LOST

Here's the part that destroys most dieters:

When you starve yourself, your metabolism slows down. But when you start eating again, your appetite returns to NORMAL levels — not reduced levels.

This means:

You return to eating the same amount

But now you burn fewer calories doing it

So you gain weight faster than before

This is not a theory — it has been proven repeatedly.

The International Journal of Obesity reported:

- 80% of dieters regain all weight lost within 1 year

- 2/3 regain MORE than they originally lost

Why?

Because:

metabolism is lower

appetite is higher

cravings are stronger

storage mode is activated

muscle mass is reduced

insulin sensitivity is lower

thyroid is suppressed

Starvation diets CREATE rebound weight gain.

Every. Single. Time.

THE MOST IMPORTANT LESSON IN THIS CHAPTER

Let me say this plainly:

Starvation is not weight loss. Starvation is delayed weight gain.

If starving yourself worked, everyone would be fit. Everyone would be healthy.

Everyone would stay lean.

But the truth is:

People who starve themselves ALWAYS rebound.

They always regain.

They always become more metabolically damaged.

And the worst part?

The rebound gets harder to fix every time.

Yo-yo dieting destroys metabolic flexibility and makes future weight loss more difficult.

The Metabolism Reset

COACH'S CORNER

I've never met a person who starved their way thin and stayed that way.

Not one.

I HAVE met people who:

- slowed their metabolism
- damaged their hormones
- wrecked their digestion
- lost muscle
- burned out
- became obsessed with food
- hated themselves
- gained weight faster than before

And every single one of them thought THEY were the problem.

They weren't.

The method failed them — not the other way around.

Starvation is a trap.

A lie.

A con.

A shortcut to nowhere.

But here's the good news:

Your metabolism CAN be repaired.

Your hormones CAN be rebalanced.

Your digestion CAN be restored.

Your appetite CAN be reshaped.

And the system to fix it isn't complicated.

It just requires feeding your body the right way.

And that's what the next chapters are going to show you.

CHAPTER 7

WHY MOST DIETS FAIL

A Breakdown of Every Popular Diet — and the Biological Reasons They Don't Produce Lasting Results

Before we dive into breaking down individual diet trends, I want to make something clear:

People don't fail diets. Diets fail people.

Every day. Every year. Every generation.

Billions of dollars are made off systems that are designed to work temporarily, collapse eventually, and bring people right back into the same cycle of desperation that made them buy in the first place.

This is not a conspiracy theory — it's business.

The diet industry profits most when:

- you lose weight fast
- regain weight faster
- blame yourself
- and start another diet

That's not a solution.

That's a trap.

This chapter explains why every popular diet works short-term — and why none of them work long-term.

And more importantly, it explains why your body was never designed for any of these systems in the first place.

THE FUNDAMENTAL LAW OF DIETING FAILURE

Before we analyze each diet individually, here is the universal truth:

Any diet that is not sustainable long-term will fail long-term.

The Metabolism Reset

It doesn't matter how much weight you lose temporarily.
It doesn't matter how motivated you are at the start.
It doesn't matter how many influencers swear by it.

If the diet is:

- restrictive
- punishing
- unsatisfying
- confusing
- stressful
- inconsistent with human biology
- mentally exhausting
- socially isolating
- physically draining

… you will NOT stick with it.

And if you don't stick with it, your body will rebound — not to your old weight, but HIGHER.

The International Journal of Obesity reports the same outcome across all restrictive diets:

- Weight lost returns within 12 months in 80% of cases
- 2/3 regain MORE than they lost
- Every cycle worsens metabolic function

This is not a failure of character.
It is a failure of strategy.

WHY EVERY DIET "WORKS" IN THE BEGINNING

Here's the uncomfortable part:
Most diets DO work — at first.
They produce:

- water loss
- rapid scale changes
- muscle loss

- glycogen depletion
- appetite suppression from stress

This creates the illusion of success.

People celebrate the early drop in weight, not realizing they're losing:

- muscle
- water
- metabolic function

NOT fat.

This early success also hooks people psychologically, which makes them ignore the early signs of metabolic damage.

But biology always wins in the end.

THE PROBLEM WITH LOW-CARB & KETO

Keto was marketed like a miracle.

The truth is more complicated.

Why people lose weight at first:

- Water loss from glycogen depletion
- Appetite suppression
- Limited food choices
- Calorie reduction without noticing
- Some improved insulin sensitivity

Why keto fails long-term:

- Extremely restrictive
- Difficult in real life
- Digestive issues
- Cravings return
- Hormonal imbalance (especially in women)
- Muscle loss without enough protein
- Gut microbiome disruption
- Rebound weight gain

The Metabolism Reset

A study in Nutrients (Paoli et al., 2013) found that keto can temporarily increase fat oxidation, but long-term adherence is extremely low.

When carbs return?

Weight rebounds faster — because metabolism slowed during restriction.

Keto doesn't fix metabolism; it bypasses it temporarily.

THE PROBLEM WITH INTERMITTENT FASTING

Intermittent fasting (IF) is one of the most misused "health trends" ever invented.

Why fasting appears to work:
- People skip meals → consume fewer calories
- Water loss
- Less snacking
- Reduced eating window

Why fasting eventually fails:
- Delayed binge eating
- Hormonal chaos (especially ghrelin and leptin)
- Cortisol spikes from long fasting windows
- Slowed thyroid function
- Reduced muscle mass
- Inconsistent hunger signals
- Difficult to sustain socially or emotionally

Studies from Obesity (2017) show that alternate-day fasting and IF produce no better long-term results than standard calorie restriction — but cause more hunger and higher dropout rates.

IF is just another form of starvation in disguise.

THE PROBLEM WITH LOW-FAT DIETS

Low-fat diets were huge in the 1980s and 1990s.
They left behind a trail of metabolic damage.

Why low-fat diets seem to work:
- Lower calorie density
- Increased carbohydrate intake temporarily suppresses appetite

Why they fail:
- Lack of essential fats harms hormones
- Increased cravings
- Elevated insulin levels
- Constant hunger
- Increased fat storage
- Poor nutrient absorption

Fat is NOT the enemy.

Overeating and under-eating are.

THE PROBLEM WITH LOW-CALORIE DIETS

(1200 calories and similar)

We covered starvation in the last chapter, but here's the summary:

Low-calorie diets ALWAYS fail because:
- The body adapts
- Metabolism slows
- Hunger increases
- Cravings increase
- Muscle is lost
- Fat is retained
- Thyroid slows
- Cortisol rises

This is the most destructive form of dieting and creates permanent metabolic dysfunction.

The "1200 calorie" myth is one of the worst pieces of misinformation in nutrition.

Most toddlers need more than 1200 calories.

THE PROBLEM WITH CLEANSES & DETOXES

Juice cleanses, detox teas, flushes, powders, 3-day resets…

Why they appear to work:

- Water loss
- Reduced bloating
- Temporary appetite suppression

Why they fail:

- Zero protein → muscle breakdown
- Blood sugar chaos
- Extreme calorie restriction
- No fiber for gut health
- Slowed metabolism
- Rapid rebound weight gain

Most "detoxes" are scams.

Your liver and kidneys detox you for free.

THE PROBLEM WITH POINTS SYSTEMS & TRACKING APPS

Weight Watchers, Noom, calorie counting apps…

Why they appear to work:

- Awareness improves eating habits
- Reduced portions
- Some structure for beginners

Why they fail long-term:

- Encourages obsession
- Encourages restriction
- Teaches people to fear food
- Doesn't fix metabolism
- Doesn't re-regulate hormones
- Doesn't improve digestion
- Often promotes processed "zero point" foods

You can't out-track a broken metabolism.

THE PROBLEM WITH "LOSE 10 POUNDS FAST" SCHEMES

Any plan that offers rapid weight loss guarantees one thing:

rapid rebound.

These diets are built on:

- dehydration
- glycogen loss
- starvation
- stimulant-based pills
- muscle cannibalization

They wreck metabolism worse than anything else.

There is no shortcut that doesn't destroy something.

WHY PEOPLE FEEL LIKE THEY "CAN'T STICK TO ANYTHING"

Here's the truth:

Almost everyone can stick to something that's:

- enjoyable
- sustainable
- consistent
- nourishing
- biologically aligned

People quit diets because diets are MISALIGNED with human biology.

Your body is not designed for:

starvation

restriction

monotony

fear of food

long fasts

cutting out entire food groups
rules so strict you break them by breathing
Your body is designed for:
rhythm
nourishment
whole food
consistency
predictable fuel
metabolic trust
The problem is not YOU.
The problem is every diet you've ever been taught.

THE DIET INDUSTRY DOESN'T WANT YOU TO KNOW THE TRUTH
There is no money in teaching people how to reset their metabolism.
There is no money in teaching people to eat consistently.
There is no money in giving people a sustainable system.
There is no money in helping people fix their hormonal environment.
But there is a LOT of money in:

- repeat customers
- rebound weight gain
- confusion
- desperation
- emotional vulnerability

Diets fail because diets are designed to fail.
But your metabolism?
That can be fixed.
And once you fix it — the diet industry loses its hold on you forever.

Leonardo Lechuga

COACH'S CORNER

I've coached people for years — regular people with jobs, kids, stress, trauma, cravings, busy schedules, and lives that don't make room for perfection.

Not one of them ever succeeded long-term on:

- keto
- fasting
- low-fat
- low-carb
- starvation
- detox teas
- points
- restriction

But EVERY SINGLE PERSON who stuck to the 2-hour whole-food method?

Their body changed.
Their mindset changed.
Their metabolism changed.
Their relationship with food changed.

Diets fail because they fight biology.
Our method works because it honors biology.

CHAPTER 8

THE METABOLISM RESET METHOD

Eat Every Two Hours. Eat Whole Foods. Eat to Heal — Not to Starve.

The first half of this book showed you what breaks metabolism.

Now we shift to what FIXES it — your system.

The Metabolism Reset Method is simple enough for anyone to follow, powerful enough to transform metabolism at any age, and sustainable enough to be a lifestyle instead of a punishment.

This chapter lays out the method step-by-step, explains the science behind every rule, and gives you the WHY behind everything your clients have already experienced.

Let's begin with what this method is not:

- It's not a diet.
- It's not calorie counting.
- It's not starvation.
- It's not cutting out entire food groups.
- It's not a "quick fix."

This is a retraining protocol for your metabolism — a biological reset that teaches your body how to burn fuel efficiently again.

And it all starts with the simplest rule:

RULE #1: EAT EVERY 2 HOURS

Timing is everything.

Let's start with the rule that scares people the most — and changes their lives the fastest.

Eat every two hours.

No skipping.

No "I'm not hungry yet."

No "I'm too busy."

Every two hours means every two hours.

WHY IT WORKS

1. It creates predictable hunger hormones.

Ghrelin fires rhythmically.

When you eat every two hours, ghrelin learns the schedule and begins sending hunger signals EXACTLY on time.

This is metabolic health.

2. It stabilizes blood sugar.

Stable blood sugar = stable insulin

Stable insulin = fat-burning mode activated.

A study in the Journal of Nutrition (2011) showed that frequent eating significantly reduces blood sugar fluctuations.

3. It stops the starvation response.

Every long gap between meals signals "danger" to your metabolism.

Every consistent meal signals "safety."

This resets metabolic trust.

4. It trains digestion.

The stomach heals itself through use — not by sitting empty for hours.

Eating every two hours:

- improves gastric emptying
- strengthens enzyme production
- reduces bloating
- increases metabolic rate

5. It eliminates binge eating.

When you're never starving, you never overeat.

This rule alone fixes decades of emotional and reactive eating habits.

RULE #2: EAT WHOLE FOODS ONLY

Real food heals. Processed food destroys.

Whole foods are foods that come from nature:

- Meat
- Eggs
- Vegetables
- Fruits
- Nuts
- Seeds
- Whole grains
- Beans
- Potatoes

Processed foods are foods that come from factories:

- chips
- crackers
- packaged snacks
- fast food
- frozen dinners
- artificial sweeteners
- refined sugar
- breaded junk
- chemical-loaded products

WHY IT WORKS

1. Whole foods have a higher thermic effect.

You burn MORE calories digesting real food.

Harvard found that whole foods can triple metabolic burn during digestion compared to processed foods.

2. Whole foods regulate hormones.

The fiber, nutrients, and natural structure activate:

- GLP-1
- Peptide YY
- Leptin

These hormones shut off cravings — naturally.

3. Whole foods digest CLEANLY.

They reduce inflammation, improve gut bacteria, and keep insulin stable.

4. Whole foods signal "abundance."

Your body interprets real food as nourishment — not survival calories.

Whole foods tell the metabolism to work harder, not conserve energy.

RULE #3: BALANCE YOUR MEALS AND SNACKS

Every meal and snack should contain:

- Protein (lean meats, eggs, yogurt, plant proteins)
- Whole-food carbs (fruit, potatoes, rice, oats)
- Healthy fats (nuts, seeds, avocados)
- Fiber (vegetables or fruit)

This isn't complicated — it's basic human nutrition.

WHY IT WORKS

1. Protein stabilizes blood sugar.

Protein slows digestion just enough to prevent crashes.

Protein also builds muscle — which boosts metabolism.

2. Whole-food carbs give steady energy.

Carbs from REAL food burn cleaner than processed carbs.

You want slow energy, not a spike-and-crash rollercoaster.

3. Healthy fats support hormones.

Your hormone system NEEDS fat to function:

- thyroid
- testosterone

- estrogen
- cortisol
- leptin
- ghrelin

No-fat diets wreck hormone balance.

4. Fiber feeds gut bacteria.

Good digestion = good metabolism.

Fiber is the fuel for the microbiome that keeps your metabolism humming.

RULE #4: NO CALORIE COUNTING

Let people breathe.

Calories do not control metabolism — hormones do.

Counting every calorie:

- increases stress
- raises cortisol
- destroys your relationship with food
- encourages starvation
- makes food the enemy
- creates obsession
- causes rebound eating
- doesn't fix metabolism

The Metabolism Reset Method focuses on:

- timing
- quality
- consistency
- hormones
- digestion

NOT numbers.

A 2018 study in JAMA found that people lost the MOST weight by focusing on whole foods — NOT calories.

RULE #5: DRINK WATER — LOTS OF IT

Hydration isn't optional.

Water supports:

- digestion
- hormone transport
- cellular repair
- thermogenesis
- mental clarity
- metabolic rate

Most people who think they're "hungry" are actually dehydrated.

When you eat every two hours, water becomes essential for nutrient transport and metabolic function.

RULE #6: GET 7–9 HOURS OF SLEEP

Sleep is where metabolism resets.

Without sleep:

- ghrelin increases
- leptin decreases
- cortisol rises
- insulin sensitivity decreases
- cravings spike

Sleep is not a luxury — it's a requirement.

This method works twice as fast with proper sleep.

RULE #7: MOVE YOUR BODY — BUT DON'T OVERTRAIN

Movement is helpful.

Overtraining is destructive.

Walking, light lifting, and mobility support metabolism.

Excessive cardio destroys it — especially when paired with low calorie intake.

The Metabolism Reset

Exercise should support your metabolism, not punish it.

RULE #8: CONSISTENCY IS KING

The metabolism responds to:

- patterns
- routines
- reliability

Not perfection.

Not extremes.

Not suffering.

If you eat every two hours for 12 days and then skip meals on day 13, your ghrelin cycle resets backwards.

The body wants stability — not surprises.

WHY THIS METHOD ALWAYS WORKS (IF YOU FOLLOW IT)

Let's recap what this system does:

Stabilizes blood sugar

Reduces insulin

Lowers cortisol

Repairs digestion

Retrains hunger hormones

Increases TEF

Protects muscle

Signals metabolic safety

Breaks binge-restrict cycles

Creates predictable hunger

Improves energy

Activates fat burning

It works because it:

- Matches human biology
- Feels natural once adapted

Leonardo Lechuga

- Builds metabolic trust
- Is sustainable
- Doesn't rely on willpower
- Doesn't require perfection
- Doesn't involve suffering
- Can be done for a lifetime

This is NOT a diet.

This is a metabolic rehabilitation program.

COACH'S CORNER

I've used this exact method with real people, in the real world, dealing with real stress, real cravings, real schedules, real trauma, and real struggles.

Not fitness models.

Not influencers.

Not people who live in the gym.

Not people with perfect discipline.

Regular people.

And every time — every single time — the body responded the same way:

It woke up.

It got hungry.

It burned fat.

It healed.

This method WORKS.

Not because it's magical, but because it aligns with how the human body was always meant to eat.

You're not breaking rules with this method.

You're returning to nature.

You're returning to biology.

You're returning to what your body has been asking for all along.

CHAPTER 9

THE 14-DAY RESET PLAN

Two Weeks to Wake Up Your Metabolism, Reset Your Hormones, and Rebuild Trust With Your Body

By now, you understand WHY your metabolism broke.

You understand WHY starvation failed.

You understand HOW eating every two hours heals your hormonal system.

Now it's time to put all of that into action.

This chapter gives you the exact 14-day protocol — the same plan I've used in real life with clients who transformed their bodies, their energy, and their entire relationship with food.

This is not a "diet."

This is not a list of foods to fear or rules to obsess over.

This is a reset manual for your biology.

Your only job for the next 14 days:

Eat real food

Eat every two hours

Stay consistent

Do that, and your metabolism will begin to fire again.

Let's break it down step-by-step.

THE STRUCTURE OF THE RESET

Every day will follow this pattern:

- Meal 1
- Snack 1
- Meal 2
- Snack 2
- Meal 3
- Snack 3

Leonardo Lechuga

That's six eating points.

You will eat every two hours, starting from your first meal of the day.

If you wake up at 7:00 a.m., your schedule might look like:

- 7:30 a.m. — Meal 1
- 9:30 a.m. — Snack 1
- 11:30 a.m. — Meal 2
- 1:30 p.m. — Snack 2
- 3:30 p.m. — Meal 3
- 5:30 p.m. — Snack 3

Adjust the hours based on your wake time — the timing matters, not the clock.

The goal is consistency, not perfection.

WHAT YOU WILL FEEL OVER THESE 14 DAYS

Let's set expectations so nothing surprises you.

DAYS 1–3 — "WHAT AM I DOING?"

- You may feel too full
- You may feel uncomfortable
- Your stomach may resist
- You may question the method
- Hunger cues feel random
- You may feel bloated or heavy

This is normal.

Your metabolism is confused and slow.

You're not broken — you're untrained.

DAYS 4–7 — "OKAY… THIS IS NOT AS BAD."

- Fullness begins to fade
- Digestion slowly wakes up

- Energy slightly improves
- Hunger starts to appear earlier
- Cravings decrease
- Mood stabilizes

Your body is adjusting.

DAYS 8–10 — "I'M STARTING TO GET HUNGRY AGAIN."

- Ghrelin (hunger hormone) is synchronizing
- Digestion speeds up
- Blood sugar stabilizes
- Less post-meal heaviness
- More consistent appetite

This is the metabolic shift preparing to happen.

DAYS 11–14 — THE METABOLIC TURNING POINT

This is where everything changes.

- Hunger appears at EXACT 2-hour intervals
- You feel lighter
- Energy lifts
- You no longer feel stuffed
- Digestion feels efficient
- Cravings drop drastically
- You might notice fat loss
- Clothes may fit differently

THIS is the moment your metabolism wakes up.

This is what we've been working toward.

If you stop now, you undo everything.

If you continue, everything gets easier from here.

THE 14-DAY PLAN: WHAT TO DO DAILY

Below is the structured plan broken into clear steps.

STEP 1: EAT WITHIN 30–60 MINUTES OF WAKING UP

This signals your metabolism:

"Wake up. Fuel is available. You are safe."

Skipping breakfast is one of the fastest ways to destroy metabolic trust.

STEP 2: EAT EVERY 2 HOURS

This is the core.

Set alarms if you must.

Use phone reminders.

Write down your schedule.

Consistency is what retrains your hormonal rhythm.

STEP 3: EACH MEAL MUST INCLUDE PROTEIN

Protein stabilizes blood sugar and supports lean muscle — the engine of your metabolism.

Examples:

- eggs
- chicken
- turkey
- Greek yogurt
- cottage cheese
- salmon
- tuna
- beans
- lentils

STEP 4: EACH SNACK MUST BE WHOLE FOOD

A "snack" does NOT mean:

- chips
- crackers

- bars
- candy
- processed junk

Snacks should be:

- fruit
- nuts
- seeds
- yogurt
- veggies + hummus
- hard-boiled eggs

Whole foods only.

STEP 5: DRINK WATER ALL DAY

Your goal:

Half your body weight in ounces per day.

Water supports digestion and hormonal balance.

STEP 6: NO PROCESSED FOODS FOR 14 DAYS

This is strict and it's important.

Processed foods:

- spike insulin
- slow digestion
- confuse hunger hormones
- increase inflammation

You're trying to heal, not harm.

STEP 7: OPTIONAL BUT POWERFUL — WALK 20–30 MINUTES DAILY

This improves insulin sensitivity and speeds up the metabolic shift.

You do NOT need heavy exercise during this reset.

EXACT MEAL & SNACK EXAMPLES (FOR ALL 14 DAYS)

These are guidelines, not a rigid menu.
Mix and match freely.

MEAL 1 OPTIONS (Breakfast)

- 2 eggs + fruit
- Greek yogurt + berries + nuts
- Oatmeal + banana + cinnamon + seeds
- Turkey sausage + scrambled egg + spinach
- Cottage cheese + pineapple

Protein + whole carb + optional fat.

SNACK 1 OPTIONS

- Apple + almonds
- Banana + peanut butter
- Greek yogurt (unsweetened)
- Hard-boiled egg
- Carrot sticks + hummus
- A handful of mixed nuts

MEAL 2 OPTIONS (Lunch)

- Chicken breast + rice + vegetables
- Salmon + quinoa + asparagus
- Turkey wrap (whole grain) + fruit
- Beef stir-fry + broccoli
- Lentils + sweet potato + greens

SNACK 2 OPTIONS

- Berries + nuts
- Cottage cheese
- Handful of cashews

- Veggies + hummus

MEAL 3 OPTIONS (Dinner)
- Chicken + potatoes + veggies
- Shrimp + brown rice
- Turkey chili
- Steak + veggies + baked potato
- Stir-fried vegetables + tofu

SNACK 3 OPTIONS (Evening)
- Greek yogurt
- Fruit + seeds
- Veggie sticks
- A small handful of nuts

This last snack prevents late-night hunger and stabilizes hormones overnight.

HOW TO TRACK YOUR PROGRESS (WITHOUT A SCALE)

You are NOT going to obsess over weight.

Weight is the LAST place metabolism shows improvement.

Here's what to pay attention to instead:

Are you hungry every 2 hours?

Do you feel less bloated?

Is your energy more stable?

Are cravings dropping?

Are you sleeping better?

Are your clothes fitting differently?

Do you feel lighter?

Is your mood more stable?

These are the REAL markers of metabolic healing.

If these are improving, the method is working —
regardless of what the scale says.

WHY THE SCALE IS MISLEADING DURING A RESET

During the first two weeks:

- You may hold water
- You may experience inflammation shifting
- Digestion is adjusting
- Muscle glycogen is replenishing
- Hormones are recalibrating

Weight can:

- go up
- go down
- stay the same

None of this matters during a reset.

The goal is metabolic rehabilitation — and that takes
time.

When your hormones align, fat loss follows
automatically.

WHAT TO DO IF YOU "MESS UP" A DAY

Let me make something crystal clear:

You cannot fail this reset unless you quit.

A bad meal doesn't break the method.

A missed snack doesn't erase progress.

A processed bite doesn't ruin everything.

This is NOT all-or-nothing.

If you slip:

- Don't punish yourself
- Don't restart the whole program
- Don't skip your next meal

- Simply get back on schedule

Consistency matters far more than perfection.

AFTER THE 14 DAYS — THE SHIFT IS PERMANENT

Once ghrelin is trained…

Once digestion is efficient…

Once insulin stabilizes…

Once cortisol drops…

Once the stomach adapts…

The system is locked in.

Your metabolism is awake.

Your hunger is predictable.

Your energy is stable.

Your body is burning fuel instead of storing it.

These two weeks change EVERYTHING.

And now you're ready to move into a sustainable long-term rhythm.

COACH'S CORNER

Listen — I've coached enough people to know the truth:

If you give me 14 days of dedication…

If you follow the timing…

If you eat real food…

If you trust the method…

If you don't quit when it feels uncomfortable…

Your body WILL respond.

Not might.

Not maybe.

Not if your genetics cooperate.

It WILL respond.

Because this system works WITH biology, not against it.

Leonardo Lechuga

Your only job?

Show up for 14 days and let your metabolism do what it was built to do.

CHAPTER 10

DO'S AND DON'TS FOR SUCCESS

The Rules, Habits, and Mindsets That Make the Metabolism Reset Work — And the Mistakes That Will Destroy It

By this point in the book, you understand WHY the Metabolism Reset works, HOW the body responds, and WHAT the 14-day plan requires.

Now we need to talk about execution — the daily habits that guarantee success, and the mistakes that stop progress dead in its tracks.

Most people don't fail because the method is hard. They fail because they make simple mistakes that undermine the entire process.

This chapter lays everything out clearly so you can avoid those traps and stay on the path.

Let's get into it.

THE DO'S OF A SUCCESSFUL METABOLISM RESET

These are non-negotiable. If you do these consistently, your metabolism WILL respond — I've seen it with every client who sticks to the plan.

DO #1: Eat Every Two Hours, No Matter What

Set alarms.

Set reminders.

Use a timer if you have to.

This rule is foundational.

Why?

- Ghrelin needs consistency
- Blood sugar needs stability
- Cortisol needs predictability
- Digestion needs rhythm

- Metabolic trust needs routine

Think of this as reprogramming your internal clock. If you skip an eating point, you interrupt that reprogramming.

DO #2: Eat Whole Foods at Every Meal
Whole foods:
- burn more calories
- digest cleaner
- stabilize blood sugar
- regulate hormones
- reduce inflammation
- rebuild metabolic trust
- eliminate cravings

Real food = real results.

DO #3: Include Protein Every Time You Eat
Protein is the foundation of metabolism.
It:
- preserves muscle
- increases thermic effect
- stabilizes blood sugar
- reduces cravings
- keeps you full
- supports thyroid hormones

Protein is the anchor of every meal.

DO #4: Hydrate Like It's Your Job
Water is required for:
- digestion
- cellular repair
- metabolism

- nutrient absorption
- hormonal function

Most people think they're hungry when they're dehydrated. Water is a cheat code.

DO #5: Plan Ahead

Failing to plan means planning to fail.

Meal prepping isn't about being perfect — it's about being ready.

Keep your fridge stocked.

Have snacks on hand.

Never rely on willpower to pick the right foods.

Preparation protects your progress.

DO #6: Pay Attention to Hunger Signals

During the first two weeks, hunger is unreliable.

But AFTER the reset?

Your hunger will come back like clockwork.

Pay attention to:

- timing
- intensity
- patterns
- feelings of fullness
- digestive changes

This is your metabolism talking to you.

Learn to listen.

DO #7: Keep It Simple

You don't need complicated recipes.

You don't need fancy ingredients.

You don't need a cookbook full of exotic meals.

Simple meals work best:

Leonardo Lechuga

- lean meat
- rice or potatoes
- vegetables
- fruit
- nuts
- yogurt

The simpler your food, the faster your metabolism heals.

DO #8: Sleep 7–9 Hours Nightly

Without sleep:

- leptin drops
- ghrelin rises
- cortisol spikes
- cravings increase
- energy drops
- metabolism slows

Sleep makes the reset work faster — and easier.

DO #9: Move Your Body Daily (Light Movement)

You don't need heavy workouts during the reset.
But you DO need movement.

- 20–30 minutes walking
- Stretching
- Mobility
- Light strength work

Movement improves insulin sensitivity and speeds the metabolic shift.

DO #10: Trust the Process

The biggest do of all.

The Metabolism Reset

Trust the science.
Trust your body.
Trust the system.
You are not guessing — you are retraining your metabolism.
This method works every time it's followed correctly.

THE DON'TS OF THE METABOLISM RESET
These are the behaviors that sabotage your progress.
Avoid them like poison.

DON'T #1: Skip Meals or Snacks
No matter how full you feel.
No matter how busy your day is.
No matter what excuses your mind throws at you.
Skipping meals sends the wrong signal:
"Food is inconsistent. Slow down."
Do NOT skip.

DON'T #2: Eat Processed Foods
Even "healthy-looking" processed foods:
- granola bars
- protein bars
- sugar-free snacks
- flavored yogurts
- frozen meals
- junk food marketed as "healthy"

Processed foods spike insulin and destroy metabolic healing.
Stick to whole, real foods.

DON'T #3: Count Calories or Obsess Over Numbers**
Calories are NOT the priority during this reset.
Hormones are.

Counting calories raises cortisol — and cortisol stalls fat loss.

Trust the structure, not the numbers.

DON'T #4: Under-Eat to "Speed Up Results"**

This one is common — and dangerous.

People think skipping meals or reducing portions will help them lose more.

Wrong.

Under-eating:

- slows metabolism
- raises cortisol
- increases fat storage
- destroys ghrelin patterns
- shuts down the thyroid

More suffering does NOT equal more results.

DON'T #5: Over-Exercise**

This is another common mistake.

People think:

"More gym = faster results."

But during a reset, too much cardio or intense training:

- increases cortisol
- increases hunger
- reduces recovery
- slows fat loss
- stresses the metabolism

Keep movement light until your metabolism is stable.

Then you can safely build intensity.

DON'T #6: Compare Yourself to Others**

Every metabolism has a different history:

- level of damage
- stress load
- sleep pattern
- dieting history
- hormone balance
- digestive health

Comparing progress is useless and demoralizing.
Your journey is YOURS.

DON'T #7: Expect Instant Fat Loss**
The reset happens internally FIRST.
Fat loss comes AFTER:
- hormone repair
- digestive improvement
- cortisol reduction
- blood sugar stabilization

The scale is the LAST place you see change.
Measure progress by:
- hunger
- energy
- mood
- sleep
- digestion
- clothing fit

Not the scale.

DON'T #8: Quit During Week One**
Week one is a test of patience — not a test of ability.
You're uncomfortable because your metabolism is healing.
This is like physical therapy for your hormones.
Don't quit before the breakthrough.

DON'T #9: Treat This Like a Temporary Diet**
This is not:
- keto
- fasting
- calorie restriction
- a detox
- a challenge
- a 30-day hack

This is a metabolic education.
It teaches you how your body wants to be fed for LIFE.

DON'T #10: Think You Can "Outsmart" Biology**
Humans try.
They always try.
"I'll just eat less."
"I'll just skip dinner."
"I'll just fast for a few days."
Your body doesn't negotiate.
If you don't respect biology, biology will humble you.
Follow the system.
Let your body win.

TROUBLESHOOTING: COMMON RESET
ISSUES & FIXES
Here are the most common problems clients report —
and how to solve them FAST.

"I feel too full."
Solution:
This is normal for the first 10 days.

The Metabolism Reset

Your stomach is reconditioning.
Keep going.

"I'm not hungry when it's time to eat."
Solution:
Eat anyway — even if it's a small amount.
Hunger will return once ghrelin resets.

"I'm craving sugar."
Solution:
Increase water intake and add fruit to snacks.
Cravings drop drastically by week two.

"I feel bloated."
Solution:
This is digestion waking up.
Walk 10 minutes after meals.

"I'm worried I'm eating too much."
Solution:
You're not.
You're eating the right AMOUNT to fix your metabolism.

"The scale went up."
Solution:
Ignore it.
It's water, glycogen, or inflammation shifting.
Not fat.

Leonardo Lechuga

COACH'S CORNER

Let me speak from experience:

Every single person who follows the do's and avoids the don'ts… succeeds.

Not some of them.

Not most of them.

ALL of them.

Your results are not about perfection.

Your results are about consistency.

This method works because it aligns with your biology — not your fears, not your diet trauma, not society's obsession with impossible standards.

Stick with the do's.

Avoid the don'ts.

Follow the rhythm.

Trust your body.

You're not dieting anymore.

You're healing.

CHAPTER 11

THE PSYCHOLOGY OF EATING

Breaking Free From Diet Culture, Food Fear, and the Mental Traps That Keep You Stuck

By now, you understand the biological side of eating — hormones, digestion, metabolism.

But there's another side that's just as powerful, and for many people, even harder to overcome:

The psychological side.

The emotional weight.

The mental conditioning.

The guilt.

The shame.

The internal war every time they look at food.

If we don't fix this, the method won't stick long-term — because the body is easy to retrain compared to the mind.

In this chapter, we're going to break down the toxic diet mindset, expose the psychological manipulation behind the weight-loss industry, and rebuild a healthy relationship with food that supports the Metabolism Reset for life.

Let's start where the damage began.

THE DIET CULTURE LIE

Most people grew up believing:

- food is the enemy
- hunger is dangerous
- fullness is shameful
- eating is emotional
- weight equals worth
- thin equals healthy
- discipline equals suffering
- restriction equals control

- success equals self-punishment

This is NOT biology.

This is conditioning — programmed into us by:

- diet companies
- social media
- magazines
- fitness influencers
- childhood experiences
- cultural expectations
- family messaging

Most people's relationships with food were broken WAY before their metabolism was.

They don't just need a metabolic reset.

They need a mental reset.

THE ALL-OR-NOTHING TRAP

This is the #1 psychological enemy of long-term success.

The mindset sounds like this:

"If I mess up a meal, the whole day is ruined."

"If I eat something bad, I might as well binge."

"I'll restart Monday."

"I already broke the diet, so who cares?"

This thinking keeps people stuck in cycles of:

- perfection → exhaustion → failure → guilt → restart

It doesn't just sabotage diets — it destroys confidence.

Here's the truth:

A single mistake only becomes a problem when you turn it into a pattern.

One bad meal doesn't break your metabolism.

But quitting? That absolutely will.

The Metabolism Reset

The Metabolism Reset works because there's no perfection required — only consistency.

You don't quit.

You continue.

You move on.

You keep the rhythm.

That's the opposite of the all-or-nothing mindset.

FOOD AS MORALITY — A PSYCHOLOGICAL PRISON

Most people have been taught to divide food into:

- "good"
- "bad"
- "allowed"
- "forbidden"
- "cheat"
- "clean"
- "dirty"

This language is toxic because it makes FOOD moral instead of BIOLOGICAL.

Now people aren't just eating food — they're judging themselves:

"I ate something bad, so I am bad."

"I messed up my diet, so I am a failure."

"I couldn't stick to it, so there's something wrong with me."

This is psychological self-destruction.

Food is not moral.

Food is not a measure of your character.

Food does not define your worth.

Food is fuel.

Food is nourishment.

Food is biology.

Leonardo Lechuga

That's it.

The moment you stop moralizing food, you free yourself from decades of guilt and shame — and you finally start to heal.

WHY STARVATION FEELS LIKE CONTROL (AND WHY IT'S A LIE)

Many people feel "powerful" when they restrict food. It feels like:

- discipline
- control
- accomplishment
- self-mastery

But this is a trap.

Restriction feels like control only in the moment. Long-term, it leads to:

- cravings
- binges
- emotional collapse
- self-blame
- obsession
- rebound weight gain

Starvation DOESN'T give you control.

It TAKES control away.

As soon as biology kicks in, the desire for food becomes overwhelming — not because you're weak, but because your body is fighting for life.

The true control comes from metabolic stability:

- predictable hunger
- predictable energy
- predictable digestion
- predictable mood

Starvation can't give you that.

Only nourishment can.

HOW DIETS CREATE FOOD FEAR

Years of restrictive dieting do something harmful:

They teach people to fear food.

Fear:

- eating too much
- eating the wrong thing
- feeling full
- being hungry
- being NOT hungry
- calories
- carbs
- fat
- eating late
- eating early
- eating at all

This fear creates cortisol spikes EVERY time you think about food.

Cortisol = fat storage.

Cortisol = cravings.

Cortisol = metabolic slowdown.

This is why many people gain weight even when eating very little — they are living in a constant state of food-related stress.

The Metabolism Reset removes food fear completely because:

- you never starve
- meals are predictable
- you're always nourished
- you never binge
- your hormones feel safe

- your body TRUSTS you

Food becomes fuel, not fear.

WHY "WILLPOWER" HAS NOTHING TO DO WITH SUCCESS

People love to blame themselves:

"I have no discipline."

"I always fail."

"I can't stick to anything."

But research is clear:

Willpower is unreliable because it's a LIMITED resource.

Stanford studies show that willpower drops when:

- you're tired
- you're stressed
- you're hungry
- you're overwhelmed
- your blood sugar is unstable

Sound familiar?

That's EVERY dieter.

Your mind is not broken.

Your willpower is not weak.

Your biology is not flawed.

The problem is the SYSTEM.

Diets require willpower — and willpower always runs out.

The Metabolism Reset doesn't require willpower.

It requires ROUTINE.

Routine is sustainable.

Routine is automatic.

Routine doesn't exhaust you.

Routine becomes natural.

That's why this method works.

EMOTIONAL EATING: IT'S NOT WHAT YOU THINK

Let's get real:

People don't emotionally eat because they're "weak."

They emotionally eat because:

- their blood sugar is unstable
- their hormones are chaotic
- cortisol is elevated
- ghrelin is firing irregularly
- leptin is unresponsive
- they're exhausted
- their body is in survival mode

In other words:

Emotional eating is often biological first, psychological second.

Once metabolism stabilizes:

- cravings drop
- emotional eating decreases
- binge urges vanish
- mental clarity improves
- stress levels lower

The emotional part becomes manageable because the biological triggers disappear.

Healing the mind starts with healing the body.

THE ROLE OF IDENTITY IN WEIGHT LOSS

This is deep — and most programs never discuss it.

Your identity controls your habits, not the other way around.

If you see yourself as:

- a dieter
- someone who always quits

- someone who struggles
- someone who can't stick to things
- someone who "messes up"

… you will always return to that identity.

But once you shift your identity to:

"I am someone who fuels my body routinely."

"I am someone who respects my biology."

"I am someone who trusts my hunger."

"I am someone who nourishes myself."

"I am someone who is consistent."

… your habits automatically align with that identity.

Identity change is the secret to long-term transformation — and the Metabolism Reset naturally creates this shift.

THE RELIEF THAT COMES FROM FOOD FREEDOM

When people finish their 14-day reset and continue into the lifestyle phase, they often say the same thing:

"Food doesn't stress me out anymore."

"I'm not afraid to eat."

"I don't binge."

"I don't crave junk like before."

"I feel normal around food."

This is not magic.

This is the result of:

- stabilized hormones
- predictable hunger
- consistent nourishment
- reduced cortisol
- improved digestion
- restored metabolic trust

The Metabolism Reset

Food becomes simple.

And simplicity is freedom.

COACH'S CORNER

Let me speak directly to you the same way I do with my clients:

You have been lied to for years — by diet culture, by society, by the fitness industry, by people who profit from your struggle.

You were never broken.

You were misled.

You were never weak.

You were starving.

You were never lazy.

Your hormones were wrecked.

You were never addicted to food.

You were trying to survive emotionally and biologically.

Once you understand the psychology behind your past behaviors, everything becomes clearer:

You weren't the problem.

The strategies were the problem.

And now you have the strategy that works WITH your biology, WITH your psychology, and WITH your real life.

This chapter is your permission slip to let go of diet trauma forever.

This is your mental reset to go with your metabolic reset.

CHAPTER 12

THE SCIENCE OF HUNGER AND FULLNESS

How Your Body Communicates, Why Diets Destroy Those Signals, and How the Metabolism Reset Restores Them

Hunger is not the enemy.

Fullness is not failure.

Cravings are not weakness.

A big appetite is not dangerous.

A small appetite is not disciplined.

These ideas came from diet culture — NOT from science, NOT from biology, and definitely NOT from anyone who understands how the human body actually works.

In fact, hunger and fullness are among the most important metabolic signals your body uses to communicate with you.

When they work properly, weight management becomes almost effortless.

When they are damaged — through dieting, fasting, stress, or processed foods — everything becomes a struggle.

This chapter teaches you what hunger really means, what fullness really means, why diets destroy both signals, and how the Metabolism Reset brings them back online.

THE TWO TYPES OF HUNGER: BIOLOGICAL VS. EMOTIONAL

Most people think hunger is simple: "I feel hungry, so I eat."

But in reality, hunger is controlled by multiple systems:

- hormones
- digestion

- stress levels
- blood sugar
- emotional triggers
- environment
- habits

To understand hunger, we must separate the two types.

TYPE 1: BIOLOGICAL HUNGER

This is genuine, physical hunger.

It is driven by hormones and body needs.

Biological hunger feels like:

- a gentle emptiness in the stomach
- a gradual increase in desire for food
- no urgency
- calm anticipation
- hunger that builds predictably
- hunger that matches your meal schedule

This is the kind of hunger healthy bodies experience — consistent, reliable, predictable.

Biological hunger is controlled by two main hormones:

Ghrelin — the hunger starter

Signals when it's time to eat.

Fires rhythmically when the body is trained.

Leptin — the hunger stopper

Signals fullness.

Controls appetite.

Regulates long-term energy balance.

When metabolism is healthy, ghrelin and leptin act like a perfect seesaw:

- Ghrelin rises → you get hungry.
- You eat.
- Leptin rises → you feel full.

- Ghrelin drops → hunger shuts off.

Simple. Clean. Beautiful biology.

TYPE 2: EMOTIONAL HUNGER

Emotional hunger is NOT about biology.

It is:

- sudden
- intense
- urgent
- specific (usually for sugar, salt, or carbs)
- tied to stress or boredom
- disconnected from physical emptiness
- followed by guilt

Emotional hunger is driven by:

- cortisol (stress)
- dopamine (reward)
- habit
- trauma
- fatigue
- loneliness
- routine

Most people don't know the difference — because dieting has confused their signals.

The Metabolism Reset fixes this.

WHY MOST PEOPLE HAVE BROKEN HUNGER SIGNALS

Before the reset, most people experience:

- hunger at random times
- no hunger in the morning
- extreme hunger at night
- feeling hungry right after a meal

- not feeling hungry all day
- craving sugar when stressed
- bingeing after skipping meals
- overeating because they feel "empty but not hungry"

This is not normal.

This is not discipline.

This is not personality.

This is metabolic dysregulation caused by:

- skipping meals
- long fasting windows
- processed food
- yo-yo dieting
- low-calorie diets
- cortisol spikes
- unstable blood sugar
- chronic stress

These habits destroy the communication between ghrelin and leptin.

HOW DIETS DESTROY GHRELIN (HUNGER)

Here's what diets do:

- skip breakfast → ghrelin misfires
- restrict calories → ghrelin becomes unpredictable
- binge at night → ghrelin shifts to evening
- eat at inconsistent times → ghrelin loses rhythm

This leads to:

- hunger at the wrong times
- no hunger when you SHOULD be eating
- low appetite during the day
- ravenous hunger at night

Leonardo Lechuga

A study in Appetite (2004) confirms that ghrelin becomes dysregulated after restrictive dieting — and takes time to repair.

This is why early in your reset, people say:

"I'm not hungry yet."
"I feel too full."

Ghrelin is literally trying to figure out what the hell is happening.

HOW DIETS DESTROY LEPTIN (FULLNESS)

Leptin resistance is one of the most damaging effects of dieting.

Low-calorie dieting causes:

- leptin levels to drop
- leptin sensitivity to decrease
- fullness signals to weaken
- hunger to increase
- cravings to intensify

A study in Nature Neuroscience found that dieting lowers leptin so dramatically that the brain perceives starvation even when body fat is normal.

This is why dieters often say:

"I never feel full."
"I'm always hungry."
"I don't know when to stop eating."

This is not lack of control —
it's hormonal damage.

THE BLOOD SUGAR CONNECTION

Blood sugar instability creates FALSE hunger.
Symptoms include:

- shakiness

- irritability
- anxiety
- sudden intense hunger
- sugar cravings
- headaches
- fatigue

This isn't real hunger.

This is the body crying out for stabilization.

When you eat every two hours, this disappears — because blood sugar never crashes.

THE ROLE OF DIGESTION IN HUNGER AND FULLNESS

Slow digestion creates fake fullness.

Fast digestion creates predictable hunger.

Before the reset, many people have:

- sluggish stomach emptying
- low enzyme production
- inflammation
- poor gut motility

After the reset:

- digestion speeds up
- gut motility improves
- bloating decreases
- hunger becomes rhythmic

This is why clients go from:

"I'm too full to eat again."

to

"I'm starving every two hours."

That shift is biological proof of metabolic improvement.

THE METABOLISM RESET: HOW IT FIXES HUNGER + FULLNESS

Let's break it down by mechanism.

1. Eating Every 2 Hours Resets Ghrelin

You eat, ghrelin drops.

Two hours pass, ghrelin rises.

Repeat this for 14 days and ghrelin becomes synchronized.

This creates:

- predictable hunger
- reduced binge eating
- improved morning appetite
- reduced nighttime hunger

This is why the two-week period is essential.

2. Whole Foods Restore Leptin Sensitivity

Processed foods damage leptin.

Whole foods repair it.

Whole-food eating reduces inflammation — which is a major cause of leptin resistance.

When leptin works, fullness works.

You feel satisfied without overeating.

3. Blood Sugar Stabilizes

Every two hours, whole-food meals prevent:

- crashes
- spikes
- cravings
- panic hunger

Stable blood sugar = stable hunger.

4. Digestion Heals

As digestion strengthens:

- meals empty faster
- hunger returns on schedule
- bloating decreases
- food breakdown improves

This increases metabolic rate AND improves hunger signals.

5. Cortisol Drops

When you stop starving:

- cortisol decreases
- stress eating reduces
- binge urges fade
- emotional hunger weakens

A relaxed body burns fat — a stressed body stores it.

THE THREE PHASES OF HEALTHY HUNGER

During the reset, hunger returns in three phases:

Phase 1: Fake Fullness

Days 1–5

Your body is confused and trying to adjust.

Phase 2: Partial Hunger Return

Days 6–10

You begin to feel lighter and hungrier at certain times.

Phase 3: Rhythmic Hunger (The Goal)

Days 10–14

Hunger arrives like clockwork every two hours.

This is the sign of metabolic health.

WHAT FULLNESS SHOULD FEEL LIKE

Fullness is NOT:

- bloated
- stuffed
- uncomfortable
- heavy
- sick

That's overeating — or poor digestion.

Healthy fullness feels like:

- calm satisfaction
- subtle closure
- the absence of hunger
- the readiness for the next eating point in two hours

Dieters often confuse "stuffed" with "full" because starvation taught them to binge.

The reset redefines fullness — gently, naturally.

CRAVINGS: WHAT THEY ACTUALLY MEAN

Cravings are not random.

They are messages.

Sugar cravings = unstable blood sugar

Salty cravings = dehydration

Carb cravings = low serotonin or fatigue

Nighttime cravings = cortisol or missed meals

Snack cravings = poor protein intake

Constant cravings = leptin dysfunction

During the reset, cravings disappear because:

- hormones stabilize
- blood sugar normalizes
- digestion improves
- whole foods regulate appetite

- cortisol decreases

Clients often say:

"I can't believe I don't crave sugar anymore."

"It's like my appetite changed."

"I don't even want junk food."

That's hormonal healing — not willpower.

COACH'S CORNER

Let me tell you like you need to hear it:

Your hunger is not broken.

Your fullness is not broken.

Your metabolism is not broken.

It's confused.

It's reacting to years of starving, dieting, stress, processed food, and mixed signals.

Your body WANTS to communicate with you.

It WANTS to feel hunger.

It WANTS to feel satisfied.

It WANTS to feel energetic.

It WANTS to burn fat.

You just need to give it the chance.

When you follow the reset, your body starts speaking clearly again:

- Hunger arrives on time.
- Fullness makes sense.
- Cravings disappear.
- Stress drops.
- Fat begins to mobilize.

This is what it feels like when your biology is finally on your side.

CHAPTER 13

UNDERSTANDING THE BODY'S FAT-BURNING SYSTEM

How Fat Storage Works, How Fat Burning Works, and Why the Reset Finally Unlocks the System Everyone Else Has Been Fighting Against

Most people think fat loss is about:

- eating less,
- burning more,
- sweating harder,
- punishing themselves,
- or finding the "perfect diet."

Wrong on all counts.

Fat loss is not guesswork.

Fat loss is not willpower.

Fat loss is not suffering.

Fat loss is a biochemical state created by the right internal environment.

If your hormones say "store fat," you will store fat.

If your hormones say "burn fat," you will burn fat.

You can't negotiate with biology.

You can only learn how to work WITH it.

This chapter explains how the fat-burning system works inside the body — and why your method reliably activates it in every client.

THE PURPOSE OF BODY FAT (IT'S NOT WHAT YOU THINK)

People treat body fat like it's some kind of moral failure, as if being overweight means you're undisciplined or weak.

But body fat exists for one reason:

Survival.

The Metabolism Reset

Fat is stored energy.

It protects you from famine.

It fuels your body when food is scarce.

It keeps your organs safe.

Fat is not the enemy — it's a safety mechanism.

The REAL problem is that modern lifestyles trick the body into storing fat even when there is no famine.

This happens because of:

- stress
- processed foods
- hormonal dysregulation
- inconsistent eating
- crash dieting
- poor sleep
- cortisol spikes
- insulin resistance

Your body THINKS it needs to store fat because you keep sending it "danger" signals.

The Metabolism Reset sends the opposite signal:

"You're safe. You're nourished. You can burn energy freely."

HOW FAT IS STORED: THE INSULIN STORY

If you learn nothing else from this chapter, learn this:

INSULIN DECIDES IF YOU STORE FAT OR BURN FAT.

That's not an opinion — that's physiology.

FACT: When insulin is high → fat burning STOPS.

FACT: When insulin is low → fat burning BEGINS.

Insulin is the body's "storage hormone."

Its job is to take excess energy and put it away for later.

Leonardo Lechuga

Insulin rises when you:

- eat sugar
- eat processed carbs
- overeat
- binge
- eat huge meals at once
- skip meals and then eat too much
- eat in long, unpredictable windows
- live stressed
- sleep poorly
- starve yourself

Starvation and bingeing both raise insulin.

Stress raises insulin.

Unstable blood sugar raises insulin.

When insulin is elevated, your body blocks access to fat stores — no matter how hard you diet, exercise, or "try."

This is why dieters lose weight only temporarily.

They reduce calories but never reduce insulin.

Your method fixes this immediately.

HOW FAT IS RELEASED: THE GLUCAGON STORY

If insulin stores fat, glucagon releases it.

Glucagon is the "fat-mobilizing hormone."

It rises when:

- blood sugar is stable
- meals are predictable
- protein intake is consistent
- stress is low
- insulin is controlled

This is EXACTLY what your Metabolism Reset accomplishes.

Your clients feel like they're burning fat "automatically" because glucagon finally has the conditions it needs to work.

This is biology — not magic.

THE ROLE OF CORTISOL: THE FAT-BLOCKING HORMONE

Cortisol is the biggest fat-loss killer next to insulin.

When cortisol is high:

- fat burning stops
- cravings spike
- insulin rises
- belly fat increases
- energy crashes
- mood becomes unstable

Cortisol increases with:

- starvation
- fasting
- high-intensity workouts
- stress
- lack of sleep
- inconsistent meals

The Metabolism Reset lowers cortisol by:

- stabilizing meal timing
- eliminating starvation cues
- improving blood sugar
- supporting sleep
- reducing stress hormones
- balancing energy intake

When cortisol drops, fat burning skyrockets.

Leonardo Lechuga

THE ROLE OF GHRELIN AND LEPTIN IN FAT LOSS

These hormones control hunger and fullness, but they also control fat mobilization.

Ghrelin (hunger hormone)

When it fires at the right times, metabolism increases.

When ghrelin misfires (due to dieting), cravings worsen and fat burning slows.

Leptin (fullness hormone)

When leptin works properly, energy expenditure increases.

When leptin is damaged, your metabolism slows to a crawl.

Diets destroy leptin.

Your method restores it.

HOW FAT ACTUALLY LEAVES THE BODY

Most people think fat "melts off" during workouts. Not true.

Most fat loss happens through breathing.

A landmark study in the BMJ (British Medical Journal) found:

- 84% of fat leaves the body as carbon dioxide
- 16% leaves as water (sweat, urine, etc.)

This means:

You burn fat when your body mobilizes it — NOT when you sweat or suffer.

Sweating is not fat loss.

Burning calories is not fat loss.

Starving is not fat loss.

Hormonal balance is fat loss.

The Metabolism Reset

WHY MOST PEOPLE NEVER ACCESS THEIR FAT STORES

Most people live in a constant fat-storage state due to:

- elevated insulin
- high cortisol
- inconsistent meal timing
- starvation behavior
- binge cycles
- processed food intake
- unstable blood sugar
- low protein intake

Their body never receives the "all clear" signal to burn stored fat.

Your method creates the PERFECT internal environment for fat burning.

THE FAT-BURNING ZONE OF THE METABOLISM RESET

Here's why your clients start losing fat around Days 10–14:

1. Ghrelin becomes regular

Hunger patterns normalize.

2. Insulin stabilizes

No more storing fat all day.

3. Cortisol drops

No stress-induced fat storage.

4. Digestion speeds up

More efficient metabolism.

5. Leptin sensitivity returns

Fullness works correctly.

6. Glucagon rises

Fat is finally released into the bloodstream.

7. Thermic effect increases

Leonardo Lechuga

Whole foods require more energy to digest.

Once these conditions align, the body begins burning fat at rest — not just during workouts.

Your clients feel:

- lighter
- warmer
- hungrier on schedule
- more energetic
- less bloated

This is the fat-burning state.

This is the metabolism waking up.

WHY FAT LOSS FEELS "EASY" AFTER THE RESET

Clients often say:

"It doesn't feel like I'm trying."

"I'm not starving."

"I'm not suffering."

"It feels natural."

"I'm hungry in a healthy way."

"I'm losing weight without dieting."

That's what happens when:

- hormones align
- digestion improves
- insulin is controlled
- cortisol drops
- leptin works
- ghrelin is predictable
- fat is accessible

Fat loss becomes a byproduct — not a battle.

This is the difference between working WITH biology versus fighting AGAINST it.

THE BIG TRUTH: YOU CAN'T FORCE FAT LOSS. YOU CAN ONLY ALLOW IT.

You cannot bully your metabolism into burning fat.

You cannot punish your body into shrinking.

You cannot starve fat away.

But you CAN create the conditions where fat burning becomes automatic.

That's what this method does.

It creates a biological environment where fat-burning hormones take over and do the work for you.

It is NOT:

- willpower
- motivation
- luck
- genetics
- suffering

It's science.

COACH'S CORNER

Here is some truth for you:

Your body isn't fighting you — it's protecting you.

It doesn't store fat to punish you.

It stores fat to keep you alive.

When you starve it, stress it, or confuse it, it panics. When you nourish it, stabilize it, and respect its timing, it relaxes.

And when the body relaxes?

It finally lets go of stored fat.

This isn't a battle.

This is cooperation.

Stop fighting your biology.

Start working with it.

Leonardo Lechuga

Your body knows exactly what to do — you just have to stop interrupting it.

CHAPTER 14

UNDERSTANDING METABOLIC DAMAGE

How Years of Stress, Dieting, Skipping Meals, and Modern Life Slow the Metabolism — and How the Reset Rebuilds It

Most people don't wreck their metabolism overnight.

It's not one bad diet.

It's not one stressful week.

It's not one month of poor eating.

Metabolic damage is death by a thousand cuts — slow, steady, cumulative changes that build up over years until eventually, the body stops responding the way it used to.

People come to me frustrated and convinced something is wrong with them:

"I barely eat and still gain weight."

"My metabolism is dead."

"Nothing works for me anymore."

"I used to lose weight easily. Now nothing moves."

They think they're broken.

They think they're weak.

They think their body has betrayed them.

But the truth is this:

Your metabolism isn't broken — it's exhausted.

This chapter explains what metabolic damage really is, how it happens, how to recognize it, and how the Metabolism Reset reverses the damage step by step.

WHAT IS METABOLIC DAMAGE?

Metabolic damage (also called metabolic adaptation or metabolic suppression) is the body's long-term reaction to:

- chronic dieting
- long gaps between meals
- starvation behavior

- high stress
- sleep deprivation
- processed foods
- inconsistent eating
- hormonal imbalance

Metabolic damage happens when the body decides:

"Food is unpredictable.

Stress is high.

I must conserve energy."

When the body senses danger, it shuts down fat burning and slows metabolism to protect you.

This is not dysfunction — it's survival.

But in the modern world, this survival mode becomes permanent.

THE 7 MAIN CAUSES OF METABOLIC DAMAGE

Let's break down the biggest culprits one by one.

1. Starvation Diets (Low-Calorie Dieting)

This is the #1 cause of metabolic suppression.

1200-calorie diets, liquid diets, extreme fasting — anything that starves the body triggers:

- slower metabolism
- hormonal imbalance
- muscle loss
- thyroid suppression
- increased fat storage

A study in the American Journal of Clinical Nutrition found that metabolism can drop by up to 30% after prolonged calorie restriction.

And here's the worst part:

The Metabolism Reset

Metabolism does NOT automatically return to normal even after you start eating again.

That's why rebound weight gain happens so fast.

2. Skipping Meals

People think skipping meals saves calories.

In reality, skipping meals:

- increases cortisol
- destabilizes blood sugar
- disrupts ghrelin rhythm
- triggers fat storage
- slows metabolic rate

Skipping meals is a metabolic landmine.

3. Eating Highly Processed Foods

Processed foods cause:

- inflammation
- insulin spikes
- leptin resistance
- unstable hunger
- gut damage

Over time, the body loses its ability to regulate appetite and metabolism properly.

4. Chronic Stress & High Cortisol

Stress is not just emotional — it's hormonal.

High cortisol:

- increases belly fat
- slows metabolism
- raises insulin
- disrupts sleep
- increases cravings

- damages digestion

You cannot burn fat in a high-cortisol state.

5. Poor Sleep

Sleep controls:

- leptin
- ghrelin
- insulin
- cortisol
- thyroid hormones

When sleep is poor, metabolism suffers.

Research in Annals of Internal Medicine shows that people who sleep less than 6 hours burn 55% less fat when dieting.

6. Inconsistent Eating Patterns

One day fasting…
One day overeating…
One day skipping breakfast…
One day bingeing at night…

This confuses hormones and teaches the metabolism not to trust your eating patterns.

Your body wants routine — not chaos.

7. Loss of Muscle Mass

Muscle is the engine of metabolism.
When you lose muscle:

- resting metabolic rate drops
- fat burning decreases
- insulin resistance increases
- rebound weight gain speeds up

The Metabolism Reset

Starvation, fasting, and aging all reduce muscle mass —
unless the diet includes protein and consistent eating.

THE SYMPTOMS OF METABOLIC DAMAGE
If you've ever felt "broken," this list will explain exactly
why.

Symptom 1: You gain weight even when eating very little
This is the classic sign of metabolic suppression.
The body is conserving energy.

Symptom 2: You are never hungry — OR always hungry
Both are symptoms of hormone imbalance.
Ghrelin and leptin are misfiring.

Symptom 3: You feel bloated all the time
Slow digestion + high cortisol = slow gastric emptying.

Symptom 4: You have low energy
Slowed metabolism reduces energy availability.

Symptom 5: You crave sugar constantly
Unstable blood sugar + cortisol = cravings.

Symptom 6: You plateau easily
Your body is operating at a reduced metabolic rate.

Symptom 7: You gain weight fast after any diet
This is a hallmark sign.
Your metabolism never recovered from previous restriction.

Symptom 8: You hold fat in the midsection

Cortisol-driven fat storage.

Symptom 9: You have sleep issues
Hormones control sleep; damaged hormones damage sleep.

Symptom 10: You feel "off" around food
Food fear, guilt, or confusion are psychological symptoms of metabolic stress.

WHY METABOLIC DAMAGE GETS WORSE WITH AGE

People love to say:

"I used to lose weight so easily when I was younger."

Yes — because:

- their hormones were stronger
- their sleep was better
- their stress was lower
- their muscle mass was higher
- they had less dieting history
- they had more metabolic flexibility

Metabolic damage accumulates.

By age 40, most people have been:

- dieting
- skipping meals
- stressed
- overeating
- undereating
- sleeping poorly
- eating processed food
- living in survival mode

for decades.

The Metabolism Reset

The Metabolism Reset reverses years of damage — not overnight, but systematically.

THE GOOD NEWS: METABOLIC DAMAGE CAN BE REVERSED

Your body is not broken.
It simply needs the right signals.
The Metabolism Reset reverses metabolic damage because it:

- stabilizes blood sugar
- lowers cortisol
- restores ghrelin rhythm
- repairs leptin sensitivity
- improves digestion
- increases thermic effect
- rebuilds metabolic trust
- preserves muscle
- increases fat access
- supports thyroid hormones

Let's break this down.

HOW THE RESET REVERSES METABOLIC DAMAGE

1. Eating Every 2 Hours Rebuilds Hormonal Rhythm
Ghrelin and leptin normalize.
Hunger becomes predictable.
Fullness becomes reliable.
This is foundational metabolic repair.

2. Whole Foods Reduce Inflammation
Inflammation is a MAJOR cause of metabolic dysfunction.

Whole foods:

- repair gut lining
- reduce bloating
- improve digestion
- stabilize insulin

This allows the metabolism to operate efficiently again.

3. Consistent Eating Lowers Cortisol

No more starvation.

No more binges.

No more erratic blood sugar.

Low cortisol = high fat-burning potential.

4. Blood Sugar Stability Repairs Insulin Sensitivity

This is crucial.

When insulin stabilizes:

- fat storage stops
- fat release increases
- cravings decrease
- energy improves

You literally unlock fat storage.

5. Protein Preserves Lean Mass

Unlike starvation diets, your reset PROTECTS muscle — which is what keeps metabolism high long-term.

6. Digestion Improves → Metabolism Improves

As the gut heals:

- nutrients absorb better
- energy increases
- metabolic rate rises

The gut and metabolism are deeply connected.

7. Sleep Improves, Reinforcing Hormonal Balance

When people nourish themselves consistently, sleep becomes deeper and more restorative.

Good sleep = powerful metabolism.

HOW LONG DOES IT TAKE TO FIX METABOLIC DAMAGE?

That depends on:

- age
- stress levels
- years of dieting
- level of hormonal imbalance
- digestive health
- sleep quality

But most people experience:

Immediate changes (Days 1–14):

- reduced cravings
- more stable energy
- less bloating
- improved clarity
- predictable hunger

Intermediate changes (Weeks 3–8):

- improved digestion
- decreased fat storage
- increased fat burning
- normalized appetite
- better sleep

Long-term changes (Months 2–6):

- sustained fat loss
- metabolic resilience
- increased muscle tone
- emotional balance around food

- strong hormonal health

You can FIX decades of damage — if you stay consistent.

THE MOST IMPORTANT LESSON IN THIS CHAPTER

Let me say this loud and clear:

If you feel like nothing has worked for you — it's not because you're broken.

It's because:

- diets destroyed your metabolism
- processed food damaged your signals
- stress blocked fat burning
- starvation weakened your hormones
- you never had a method that aligned with biology

Your body WANTS to heal.
Your metabolism WANTS to work.
Your hormones WANT to balance.
Your hunger cues WANT to return.

The moment you stop fighting your biology and start feeding it correctly — everything changes.

COACH'S CORNER

Don't be discouraged:

Most of the people I've coached came to me feeling defeated.
They had tried everything.
They thought they had "slow metabolism," "bad genetics," or "no discipline."

The Metabolism Reset

But once they followed the reset — once they put real fuel in their body, every two hours, with whole foods — something amazing happened:

Their metabolism came back.

Their hunger returned.

Their energy rose.

Their cravings disappeared.

Their body finally responded.

You are NOT too old.

You are NOT too damaged.

You are NOT too far gone.

Your metabolism is waiting for the right environment — and once you create that environment, your body will transform.

CHAPTER 15

HOW TO MAINTAIN YOUR RESULTS AFTER THE RESET

The Lifestyle Phase: Living Lean, Energized, and Metabolically Active for Life

You've reset your metabolism.

You've rebuilt your hunger signals.

You've restored hormonal balance.

You've gotten predictable hunger, steady energy, and a stable mood.

Your body is burning fat instead of storing it.

Now comes the most important part:

Staying in the metabolic sweet spot for life.

The 14-Day Reset is like physical therapy for your metabolism.

It repaired the damage.

It fixed the communication.

It restored the rhythm your body needed.

But long-term success requires understanding:

- what habits to KEEP
- what habits can RELAX
- what habits you can PERSONALIZE
- and what habits you should NEVER abandon

This chapter is about transitioning from the "reset phase" into the "lifestyle phase" — where this becomes effortless… and enjoyable.

Let's dive in.

THE GOAL OF THE LIFESTYLE PHASE

The Lifestyle Phase has three goals:

1. Keep the metabolism active

2. Maintain hormonal balance

3. Create a life you can sustain forever

The Reset was the foundation.

The Lifestyle Phase is the house you live in.

And unlike every diet you've ever tried, this lifestyle doesn't feel restrictive.

It feels natural — because it matches your biology.

HOW OFTEN SHOULD YOU EAT AFTER THE RESET?

Here is the truth:

You do NOT need to eat every 2 hours forever.

The 2-hour rhythm is the healing phase.

Once your hormones are stable and your hunger patterns are predictable, you can transition to a flexible schedule that still keeps your metabolism strong.

I recommend one of these long-term structures:

OPTION 1: Every 3 Hours (Most Popular Long-Term Plan)

Meal

Snack

Meal

Snack

Meal

This keeps hormones stable while giving more flexibility.

Great for:

- busy schedules
- work environments
- gym-goers
- parents
- normal daily life

OPTION 2: Every 2–4 Hours (Flexible Pattern)
This lets your hunger guide you.
You'll find your body naturally asks for food once your rhythm is restored.
This is metabolic freedom.

OPTION 3: Stay at Every 2 Hours (For Those With Heavy Damage)
Some people feel best at 2 hours long-term:
- individuals with past eating disorders
- people who chronically under-ate
- people with extreme metabolic damage
- athletes who need consistent fuel

There is no shame in staying at 2 hours — it's not "extra."
It's smart for people who need more support.

THE 4 HABITS YOU MUST KEEP FOR LIFE
These are non-negotiable.
If you abandon these, your metabolism WILL slide backward.
Let's break them down.

HABIT #1: Eating Whole Foods 80–90% of the Time
Whole foods heal.
Processed foods inflame.
You don't need to be perfect — you need to be consistent.
Aim for:
- lean proteins
- vegetables
- fruits

- whole grains
- potatoes
- nuts & seeds

Whole foods keep your hormones balanced.

HABIT #2: Never Letting Yourself Get Ravenously Hungry

Letting hunger get extreme triggers:

- cortisol spikes
- cravings
- overeating
- blood sugar crashes
- metabolic stress

You don't have to eat by the clock anymore…
but you DO have to respect your biology.

Eat before you're starving, not after.

HABIT #3: Eating Protein With Every Meal

Protein is still the anchor.

It keeps:

- metabolism high
- hunger regulated
- muscle preserved
- cravings low

Protein = stability.

This is not up for debate.

HABIT #4: Hydration (Every Single Day)

Water assists:

- metabolism
- digestion
- hunger signals

- hormones
- fat mobilization

Dehydration is one of the fastest ways to throw off your hunger cues and blood sugar.

Make hydration part of your identity.

THE 4 HABITS YOU CAN RELAX (AFTER THE RESET)

These habits were essential during the Reset…
but after recovery, you have flexibility.

HABIT TO RELAX #1: Strict 2-Hour Timing

Once your hunger rhythm returns:

Your body will guide you.

If hunger hits at 2 hours → eat.
If hunger hits at 3 hours → eat.
If hunger hits at 4 hours → eat.

The principle:

Eat when your body asks, not when diet culture demands.

HABIT TO RELAX #2: No Evening Snacks

During the Reset, evening snacks helped keep hormones stable overnight.
After the Reset, you can listen to your hunger:

- If you're hungry → eat a small whole-food snack
- If you're not → skip it guilt-free

The rule:

Honor your biology, not the clock.

HABIT TO RELAX #3: Limited Food Variety

The Metabolism Reset

During the Reset, simplicity = metabolic healing.
Now you can expand your menu without fear:

- more spices
- more homemade recipes
- more variety
- more cultural foods
- more flavor

Just don't return to processed options.

HABIT TO RELAX #4: Minimal Exercise
In the Reset, we avoided over-training.
In the Lifestyle phase, movement becomes a superpower.
More on that soon.

HOW TO HANDLE TREATS WITHOUT RUINING METABOLISM
This is where people fear they will "fall off."
Let me be clear:
Treats don't break metabolism.
Patterns do.
Here's how to enjoy food without undoing your progress:

Rule #1: Never eat treats on an empty stomach.
If insulin spikes while you're in a depleted state → FAT STORAGE.
If you eat a treat after protein + fiber → controlled insulin, minimal damage.
Protein first, treat second.
This alone saves your metabolism.

Rule #2: Treats should be the exception, not the routine.
Aim for:

- 1–3 treat meals per week
- NOT 1–3 treat days

Big difference.

Rule #3: No guilt. Ever.
Guilt raises cortisol.
Cortisol raises insulin.
Insulin stores fat.
Your guilt is more damaging than the food.

Rule #4: Get back to normal at the next meal.
Not tomorrow.
Not next week.
Not "after you punish yourself."
Just go right back to your normal eating rhythm.
This prevents spirals.

HOW TO TRAVEL AND STAY ON TRACK
Travel does NOT have to destroy your reset results.
Here's how to keep everything stable:

Travel Rule #1: Always pack whole-food snacks.
Examples:

- nuts
- fruit
- beef sticks (clean ingredients only)
- hard-boiled eggs
- clean protein bars (minimal ingredients)

Never let airports or gas stations decide your
metabolism.

Travel Rule #2: Eat every 3 hours — NOT every 2

Travel is stressful.
Give yourself flexibility.

Travel Rule #3: Hydrate aggressively
Travel dehydrates you → raises cortisol → increases cravings.
Keep your metabolism calm with water.

HOW TO HANDLE SOCIAL EVENTS

Social events used to throw people off.
Not anymore.
Follow these steps:

1. Eat protein before the event
Reduces cravings and protects blood sugar.

2. Survey the food — make a plan
Pick your plate with intention.

3. Prioritize whole foods where possible
Meat, fruit, vegetables first.

4. Treats? Enjoy them — but not blindly
You're not a prisoner.
You're in control now.

EXERCISE IN THE LIFESTYLE PHASE

During the Reset, we avoided intense workouts because the metabolism was recovering.
But once the metabolism is stable?
Exercise becomes a multiplier.
The best long-term training combination:

- Strength training (3–4 days/week) builds muscle → increases metabolism
- Walking (daily) reduces cortisol → improves fat burning
- Optional: HIIT (1–2 days/week) ONLY if stress is low and sleep is good

Remember:

Exercise should support metabolism — not replace proper eating.

THE ONE THING THAT WILL DESTROY YOUR RESULTS

Let me be brutally honest:

Going back to skipping meals WILL ruin everything.

Skipping meals:

- raises cortisol
- destabilizes blood sugar
- shuts down fat burning
- reverses ghrelin rhythm
- triggers binges
- rebuilds metabolic distrust

Your metabolism CANNOT thrive without consistent fuel.

This is the single most important thing to avoid.

WHAT SUCCESS LOOKS LIKE IN THE LIFESTYLE PHASE

Here's what you'll notice:

- steady, natural hunger
- consistent energy all day
- better sleep
- fewer cravings

- easier weight maintenance
- slow, steady fat loss
- no guilt around food
- normal social eating
- stable mood
- sustainable habits

This is what life is supposed to feel like.

COACH'S CORNER

So now what:

You didn't come this far just to go back to the old habits that damaged your metabolism in the first place.

You earned this new body.

You earned this new energy.

You earned this freedom.

The Lifestyle Phase is where the real transformation happens — not because you're trying harder, but because you're finally living in alignment with how your body was created to function.

You don't need to be perfect.

You just need to be consistent.

You don't need to suffer.

You just need to nourish.

You don't need to restart anymore.

You just need to LIVE this.

This is not a diet.

This is who you are now.

CHAPTER 16

THE ROLE OF MOVEMENT: TRAINING FOR A HIGH METABOLISM

How to Move, How Often to Move, and Why Movement Matters More Than "Working Out" When It Comes to Long-Term Fat Burning

Most people think fat loss happens in the gym.

It doesn't.

Fat loss happens through:

- stable hormones
- balanced blood sugar
- strong digestion
- consistent eating
- stress management
- recovery
- daily movement

The gym can support fat loss — but it cannot create it.

In fact, the way most people work out actually slows fat loss because they:

- train too hard
- train too often
- raise cortisol
- eat inconsistently
- don't recover
- treat training like punishment

The truth is:

Exercise should never replace nutrition — it should amplify it.

This chapter shows you how to move your body in a way that increases metabolism, protects hormones, and makes fat loss easier than ever before.

THE DIFFERENCE BETWEEN MOVEMENT AND EXERCISE

Before we go deeper, you need to understand this distinction:

Movement = metabolic maintenance

Walking

Stretching

Standing more

Light activity

Daily non-exercise activity

Movement reduces stress, lowers cortisol, and keeps fat burning active all day.

Exercise = metabolic stimulus

Strength training

Cardio

HIIT

Sports

Classes

Exercise challenges the body and builds strength — but it also raises cortisol.

Both are important.

But one is for health, and the other is for progress.

Most people rely ONLY on exercise and ignore movement — and that's why they struggle.

WHY MOVEMENT (NOT "WORKING OUT") IS THE REAL FAT-BURNING SUPERPOWER

NEAT (Non-Exercise Activity Thermogenesis) — which is the energy you burn through daily movement — accounts for hundreds more calories burned than any gym session.

Examples of NEAT:

- walking

- taking stairs
- cleaning
- cooking
- yard work
- standing
- casual moving

Studies show that NEAT:

- improves insulin sensitivity
- reduces cortisol
- increases fat utilization
- stabilizes hormones
- increases daily caloric burn

This is why people who walk 8–12k steps daily stay lean without restrictive diets.

Movement = metabolism.

WHY THE RESET LIMITS INTENSE EXERCISE (THE SCIENCE)

During the Reset Phase, intense exercise is limited for 3 reasons:

1. Hard training raises cortisol

Cortisol blocks fat loss.

Your metabolism cannot heal in high stress.

2. Hard training increases hunger dysregulation

When hormones are already unstable, exercise makes hunger unpredictable.

3. Hard training increases inflammation

The gut and hormones need to calm down during the reset.

This is why your method works so consistently — it fixes the internal system FIRST.

Once the metabolism is stable, THEN exercise becomes a superpower.

THE BEST TYPE OF TRAINING FOR METABOLIC HEALTH: STRENGTH TRAINING

If you want the biggest long-term metabolic payoff, nothing beats building muscle.

Muscle:

- burns more calories at rest
- improves insulin sensitivity
- increases metabolic flexibility
- reduces fat storage
- supports hormonal balance
- strengthens bones
- improves posture and mobility

A study in Sports Medicine found that strength training increases resting metabolic rate for up to 72 hours after each session.

Strength training literally turns your body into a better fat-burning machine.

THE THREE PILLARS OF METABOLIC TRAINING

To train for a high metabolism, combine:

Pillar 1: Strength Training (3–4 Days/Week)
Focus on:

- squats
- deadlifts
- presses
- rows

- lunges
- hip hinges

These are compound movements that train multiple muscles at once — giving you maximum metabolic return.

Rep ranges can vary:

- 8–12 reps for muscle building
- 12–20 reps for metabolic conditioning

You do NOT need heavy weights to get results — you need consistency.

Pillar 2: Walking (Daily)

Walking is the most underrated fat-loss tool on Earth.

Walking:

- lowers cortisol
- stabilizes blood sugar
- reduces cravings
- improves digestion
- burns fat directly
- supports hormone balance

You should aim for at least:

- 7,000 steps per day minimum
- 10,000–12,000 for accelerated results

Walking also improves mental health and sleep — both crucial for metabolism.

Pillar 3: Optional HIIT (1–2 Days/Week)

High-intensity training is powerful — but only when:

- sleep is good
- stress is low
- hormones are stable
- recovery is strong

HIIT increases:

- fat oxidation
- metabolic conditioning
- cardiovascular health

BUT it also increases cortisol temporarily.

This is why HIIT must be earned, not forced.

If your lifestyle is stressful, HIIT is optional — not mandatory.

THE BIGGEST EXERCISE MISTAKES THAT RUIN METABOLISM

Let's expose the common errors:

Mistake #1: Too much cardio

Hours of cardio per week:

- increases cortisol
- reduces muscle
- slows metabolism
- increases cravings
- stalls fat loss

Cardio should supplement strength training — not replace it.

Mistake #2: Training on an empty stomach

This is one of the FASTEST ways to kill metabolism.

Training fasted raises cortisol dramatically and teaches the body to:

burn muscle instead of fat.

Eat something small (protein + carbs) before training.

Mistake #3: Treating exercise like punishment for food

Exercise should never be used to "cancel out" calories.

This behavior:

- destroys mental health
- increases cortisol
- encourages binge-restrict cycles
- damages metabolism

Exercise is a privilege — not punishment.

Mistake #4: Working out too intensely too often

Your body cannot burn fat if it is constantly in recovery mode.

Fat loss requires:

- rest
- nourishment
- recovery
- hormonal stability

Not nonstop grind.

Mistake #5: Inconsistency

Working out hard for 2 weeks and then disappearing for 3 months doesn't work.

Consistency beats intensity 100 times out of 100.

HOW TO STRUCTURE YOUR LONG-TERM TRAINING WEEK

Here is the ideal formula for a high-metabolism lifestyle:

OPTION A: Balanced Weekly Plan

Monday: Strength

Tuesday: Walk

Wednesday: Strength

Thursday: Walk

Friday: Strength

The Metabolism Reset

Saturday: Optional HIIT or Walk
Sunday: Recovery Walk + Stretch

OPTION B: Beginner-Friendly Plan
Monday: Full-body strength
Wednesday: Light strength + walk
Friday: Full-body strength
Daily: Walk

OPTION C: Advanced Plan
Mon: Legs + Walk
Tue: Upper + Walk
Wed: HIIT + Walk
Thu: Lower + Walk
Fri: Upper + Walk
Sat: Hike/Long Walk
Sun: Rest

No matter the plan:
Walking remains non-negotiable.

THE ROLE OF MOBILITY, FLEXIBILITY &
RECOVERY

Most people ignore recovery, and that costs them results.
Recovery includes:

- stretching
- foam rolling
- warm-ups
- cool-downs
- hydration
- sleep

These activities:

- lower cortisol
- improve muscle function
- reduce inflammation
- help prevent injury
- improve metabolic rate

Remember:

Fat burning happens during recovery, not during the workout.

THE CONNECTION BETWEEN MOVEMENT & HORMONES

Movement improves:

Insulin sensitivity

Your cells respond better → less fat storage.

Cortisol balance

Walking lowers stress → more fat burning.

Leptin signaling

Your fullness cues strengthen.

Thyroid function

Your metabolic engine stays strong.

Digestive motility

Food moves better → less bloating.

Movement is hormonal therapy — not just fitness.

HOW TO KNOW YOU ARE TRAINING FOR METABOLIC HEALTH

Signs your movement routine is working:

- you have steady energy
- you're hungrier on a predictable rhythm
- sleep improves
- cravings decrease
- body composition changes

- digestion improves
- mood increases
- workouts feel enjoyable, not exhausting

This is what metabolic alignment looks like.

COACH'S CORNER

Working out is not the key.

Movement is.

Sweating isn't the goal — consistency is.

Punishing your body isn't the goal — building it is.

Starving yourself isn't the goal — fueling yourself is.

You don't need to train like an athlete to get lean.

You don't need to destroy yourself in the gym to burn fat.

You don't need to be perfect — you just need to move.

Your metabolism doesn't care how fancy your workout is. It cares that your hormones are balanced, your meals are consistent, your stress is low, and your daily movement is steady.

Move your body.

Build your muscle.

Walk every day.

Respect your biology.

Do that…

and you will have a high metabolism for the rest of your life.

CHAPTER 17

HOW TO REIGNITE YOUR METABOLISM AFTER A SETBACK

The 24-Hour, 48-Hour, and 7-Day Recovery Protocols for Getting Back on Track Without Starting Over or Losing Progress

Let's get something straight:

Setbacks don't ruin your metabolism — quitting does.

Every single person has moments where they:

- overeat
- skip meals
- binge during stress
- go on vacation
- eat processed foods
- drink alcohol
- fall off the rhythm

Life happens.

Perfection doesn't exist.

And honestly?

It's not supposed to.

Your metabolism is not fragile.

Your hormones are not glass.

Your progress is not erased because of a weekend, a birthday, a trip, or a rough week.

The key is knowing how to recover the right way — without panic, punishment, guilt, or starting over from scratch.

This chapter shows exactly how to get back into alignment FAST.

THE MOST IMPORTANT RULE: DON'T PANIC

When people slip, their first instinct is usually:

- "I messed everything up."
- "My metabolism is ruined."
- "I have to start all over."
- "I need to starve myself tomorrow."
- "I need to train extra hard."

Wrong.
Wrong.
Wrong.
And VERY wrong.

Panic leads to one of two dangerous responses:

1. Starve yourself the next day

Raises cortisol → slows metabolism → increases hunger → leads to bingeing.

2. Punish yourself with excessive exercise

Raises cortisol → increases cravings → disrupts digestion → hurts recovery.

Both responses do MORE metabolic damage than the slip itself.

The correct response is calm, normalcy, and biological consistency.

WHY SETBACKS FEEL WORSE THAN THEY ARE

A setback doesn't damage your metabolism.
But the mental reaction to it can.

What makes people spiral isn't the food — it's:

- guilt
- shame
- fear
- perfectionism
- negative self-talk
- "I blew it so I may as well keep going"

This all-or-nothing thinking is diet culture's poison.

You're not doing that anymore.

From now on, setbacks are handled scientifically — not emotionally.

THE 24-HOUR METABOLIC RESET (THE NEXT DAY PROTOCOL)

This is your go-to method for the day AFTER overeating or missing meals.

This simple routine pulls your metabolism back into alignment FAST.

Step 1: Hydrate First Thing in the Morning (16–24 oz)

Overeating — especially processed foods — increases inflammation and water retention.

Hydration:

- flushes excess sodium
- decreases bloating
- jumpstarts digestion
- lowers cortisol

This is non-negotiable.

Step 2: Eat a Protein-Rich Breakfast (No Skipping)

Skipping meals the morning after overeating is one of the worst mistakes.

Eating breakfast:

- stabilizes blood sugar
- reestablishes ghrelin rhythm
- reduces cravings later
- prevents binge-restrict cycles

Examples:

- eggs + fruit
- Greek yogurt + berries

- chicken + veggies
- protein shake + banana

Step 3: Return to Your Eating Rhythm (Every 2–3 Hours)

The key is NOT restricting.

The key is:

returning your hormones to their normal pattern.

Normalizing your eating rhythm:

- lowers cortisol
- regulates ghrelin
- restores leptin
- stabilizes insulin

This is metabolic recovery.

Step 4: Whole Foods Only (for 24 Hours)

After processed food, the body needs clean fuel.

Whole foods reduce inflammation quickly.

Focus on:

- meat
- vegetables
- fruit
- potatoes
- rice
- nuts
- eggs

No "detox."

No starvation.

Just clean, steady nourishment.

Step 5: A 20–30 Minute Walk After Dinner

Walking lowers blood sugar naturally and supports digestion.

It helps:

- reduce cravings
- improve sleep
- stabilize hormones
- accelerate fat recovery

This step is powerful.

THE 48-HOUR EXTENDED RECOVERY (FOR BIGGER SETBACKS)

If you've had a weekend or multi-day slip — alcohol, heavy meals, travel — the 48-hour protocol is perfect.

Here's what to do:

Day 1 (Follow the 24-Hour Protocol)

Return to rhythm.

Drink water.

Eat whole foods.

Walk.

Day 2: Add Light Movement + Increase Protein

The goal is NOT to burn calories — it's to lower cortisol and restore stability.

Recommended Day 2 moves:

- walking
- stretching
- yoga
- light strength training
- mobility work

Avoid:

- high-intensity workouts
- long cardio sessions
- anything that spikes cortisol

The Metabolism Reset

Protein intake increases fullness and stabilizes blood sugar. Add:

- an extra serving of protein
- Greek yogurt
- a protein shake

This improves leptin balance.

THE 7-DAY RAPID REALIGNMENT (WHEN YOU FEEL "WAY OFF")

This is for people who feel completely derailed:

- digestive system off
- cravings out of control
- sleep disrupted
- bloating constant
- sugar intake high
- low energy
- inconsistent eating
- emotional eating

The 7-Day Realignment is NOT a punishment. It's a metabolic tune-up.

Here's how it works:

Days 1–2: Follow the 24-Hour + 48-Hour Protocols
Establish stability.

Days 3–4: Eat Every 2 Hours (Mini Reset)
Return briefly to the original reset rhythm.
This:

- reestablishes hunger cues
- repairs digestion
- stabilizes insulin
- lowers cortisol

- reduces cravings

Days 5–7: Phase Back to Every 3 Hours
Transition out gently.
This protects your metabolism and prevents binge cycles.

THE GOLDEN RULE OF SETBACK RECOVERY
Let me make this absolutely clear:
You do NOT start the entire 14-day reset over.
Why?
Because:
- the damage is not erased
- hormones don't go back to zero
- metabolism doesn't "reset backward"
- you didn't undo your progress

Setbacks are speed bumps — not restarts.
Diet culture brainwashed people into believing:
"You messed up. Start all over."
Not anymore.
Now we respond with science — not shame.

HOW TO HANDLE SPECIFIC TYPES OF SETBACKS
Here are common real-life scenarios and exactly what to do.

Scenario 1: You Ate a Huge Dinner or Dessert
Use the 24-hour protocol.
Do NOT restrict.

Scenario 2: You Skipped a Whole Day of Eating

The Metabolism Reset

Get back to rhythm immediately.

Eat every 2 hours for the next 24 hours.

This repairs ghrelin.

Scenario 3: You Binged at Night

Eat breakfast normally.

Hydrate.

Return to rhythm.

Night binges are cortisol-driven — stability fixes them.

Scenario 4: You Went on Vacation

Use the 48-hour protocol when you get home.

Do NOT punish yourself.

Scenario 5: You Overdrank Alcohol

Hydrate heavily.

Whole foods only for 24–48 hours.

Prioritize sleep.

Add gentle walking.

Alcohol dehydrates → raises cortisol → destabilizes blood sugar.

Water + consistency fix it.

Scenario 6: You Fell Off for Weeks

Use the 7-Day Realignment.

Not the full reset (unless you want the full structure).

Your body remembers what you taught it — you just need to remind it.

THE MINDSET OF A METABOLICALLY HEALTHY PERSON

The person with a strong metabolism thinks differently:

- "A setback is just data."
- "I fuel my body, not punish it."
- "I know how to recover fast."
- "My lifestyle doesn't fall apart because of one choice."
- "I trust my hunger signals."

This mindset makes you unstoppable.

COACH'S CORNER

Look — life is going to life.

You're going to have holidays, vacations, stressful days, celebrations, rough nights, weekends with friends, and moments where things get out of rhythm.

That doesn't mean you failed.

That doesn't mean you're starting over.

That doesn't mean everything is ruined.

You're not a dieter anymore.

You're someone who understands your metabolism.

You're someone who knows how to recover.

You're someone who feeds their body with purpose.

You're someone who doesn't panic when life gets messy.

You've got tools now.

You've got knowledge now.

You've got control now — REAL control, not diet control.

Setbacks don't define you.

Your comeback does.

CHAPTER 18

THE HORMONAL BLUEPRINT

Understanding Female & Male Metabolism Differences — And How to Tailor the Reset for Each Body

Men and women can eat the same foods, follow the same plan, and live the same lifestyle…

but get completely different results.

That's not failure.

That's not lack of discipline.

That's not laziness.

That's biology.

Hormones determine:

- how easily you lose fat
- where you store fat
- how hungry you feel
- how you respond to stress
- how much muscle you can build
- how food affects your body
- how consistent your metabolism stays
- how cravings show up
- how energy fluctuates
- and even how motivated you feel

This chapter will teach you how male and female hormones differ, how they each impact metabolism, and how the Metabolism Reset works uniquely for both.

THE BIG PICTURE: MEN VS. WOMEN IN METABOLISM

Women burn fewer calories at rest on average.

Women store more fat biologically.

Women experience more hormonal fluctuations.

Women have higher cortisol sensitivity.

Women have a more complex relationship with hunger cues.

Women gain fat faster under stress.

Women lose fat slower under stress.

Men, meanwhile:

- lose weight faster
- build muscle faster
- burn calories more efficiently
- have lower cortisol sensitivity
- have higher testosterone
- have simpler hormonal patterns

It's not unfair — it's evolution.

And once you understand these differences, you stop fighting biology and start working with it.

SECTION 1: THE FEMALE METABOLIC BLUEPRINT

Women aren't "bad" at dieting.

Women aren't "too emotional."

Women aren't "inconsistent."

Women are hormonally complex — period.

Their metabolism is influenced by:

- estrogen
- progesterone
- testosterone
- cortisol
- thyroid hormones
- insulin
- leptin
- ghrelin

And these hormones shift constantly throughout the menstrual cycle, pregnancy, postpartum, and especially menopause.

Let's break it down.

ESTROGEN — THE FEMALE METABOLIC SUPERPOWER

Estrogen is powerful.

When balanced, it:

- improves insulin sensitivity
- enhances fat burning
- reduces appetite
- boosts serotonin
- increases mood stability
- protects metabolism
- improves muscle tone

When low or high, it causes:

- cravings
- fat storage
- mood swings
- poor sleep
- bloating

Estrogen is the reason:

Women lose fat easiest in the first half of their cycle.

PROGESTERONE — THE APPETITE HORMONE

Progesterone rises in the second half of the cycle.

High progesterone can:

- increase hunger
- increase cravings
- slow digestion
- increase water retention

- lower insulin sensitivity

This is why women often feel:

- hungrier
- more tired
- more bloated
- more "puffy"

during the PMS phase.

It's not weakness.

It's hormones doing their job.

TESTOSTERONE IN WOMEN

Women have testosterone too — just less of it.

Healthy testosterone:

- increases lean muscle
- boosts metabolism
- increases energy
- improves fat burning
- supports libido

Low testosterone in women often causes:

- stubborn fat
- low energy
- decreased motivation
- reduced muscle
- slow metabolism

Crash dieting DESTROYS testosterone levels in both sexes, but especially women.

The Metabolism Reset repairs this.

THE MENSTRUAL CYCLE AND METABOLISM

Let's break this down simply.

Week 1: Menstrual Phase (Day 1–5)

The Metabolism Reset

Low estrogen, low progesterone.
Energy is low.
Hunger is moderate.
Carb tolerance is lower.
Women should eat:

- whole foods
- high protein
- moderate carbs
- lots of hydration

Movement: walking + light training.

Week 2: Follicular Phase (Day 6–14)
Estrogen rises — metabolism improves.
Women feel:

- stronger
- leaner
- less hungry
- more energetic
- more insulin sensitive
- better mood

This is the BEST fat-burning window of the month.
Movement: heavier training works great here.

Week 3: Ovulation (Day 14–16)
Estrogen peaks.
Women feel:

- strong
- sexy
- confident
- energetic

This is another great fat-burning window.
Movement: great time for strength training.

Week 4: Luteal Phase (Day 17–28)

Progesterone increases.

Women feel:

- hungrier
- slower digestion
- cravings
- water retention
- mood shifts

This is NORMAL.

Women need:

- more calories
- more whole-food carbs
- more protein

Trying to "diet harder" during PMS makes cravings WORSE.

WHY WOMEN LOSE WEIGHT SLOWER (AND WHY IT'S NORMAL)

Women store fat more easily because:

- estrogen protects fertility
- progesterone increases appetite
- cortisol sensitivity is higher
- women retain more water
- women burn fewer calories at rest

This is biology — not failure.

Women lose weight slower...

BUT they KEEP it off more reliably once hormones are stable.

That is the result of metabolic healing — not dieting.

SECTION 2: THE MALE METABOLIC BLUEPRINT

Men have a simpler hormonal profile.

The dominant hormones are:

- testosterone
- cortisol
- insulin
- thyroid hormones

Let's break it down.

TESTOSTERONE — THE MALE SUPERPOWER

Men have 10–20x more testosterone than women.

Testosterone:

- increases muscle
- boosts metabolism
- increases fat burning
- stabilizes mood
- improves energy
- increases insulin sensitivity

This is why:

Men lose fat MUCH faster than women.

Men gain muscle MUCH faster than women.

It is not effort.

It is not discipline.

It is not "working harder."

It is testosterone.

Crash dieting kills testosterone — which is why men who starve themselves often regain fat rapidly afterward.

The Metabolism Reset protects and restores testosterone.

CORTISOL IN MEN

Men tolerate stress better hormonally, but when cortisol gets chronically high it leads to:

- belly fat
- low testosterone
- inflammation
- low motivation
- sleep disruption

Men ALSO need metabolic healing — they simply respond faster.

INSULIN & MEN

Men are more insulin sensitive than women on average. This means:

- men burn carbs better
- men store less fat from carbs
- men handle overeating differently
- men recover from slips faster

But LONG-TERM overeating harms men significantly, especially around the waistline.

THE DIFFERENCES THAT MATTER MOST

Let's summarize the critical points:

1. Women lose weight slower, but more permanently

Once hormones stabilize, women's bodies become extremely efficient.

2. Men lose weight faster due to testosterone

But regain quickly if dieting destroys hormone balance.

3. Women need more consistency

Their hormones fluctuate more.

4. Men need more muscle stimulus

Strength training boosts their testosterone and metabolism.

5. Women need more whole-food carbs during PMS
This reduces cravings and stabilizes mood.

6. Men tolerate more exercise stress
But can overtrain if meals are skipped.

HOW TO OPTIMIZE THE METABOLISM RESET FOR WOMEN

Women benefit from these additions:

1. Increase complex carbs during PMS
Potatoes, fruit, rice, oats.
Reduces cravings and stabilizes mood.

2. Reduce HIIT during luteal phase
Too much intensity raises cortisol.

3. Prioritize protein during menstrual cycle
Improves energy and reduces cravings.

4. Don't fear hunger fluctuations
Hunger WILL shift throughout the month — that's normal.

5. Keep consistency higher
Women thrive with routine.

HOW TO OPTIMIZE THE RESET FOR MEN
Men benefit from:

1. Strength training 3–4x per week

Testosterone booster.

2. More total calories
Men burn more — they need more fuel.

3. Higher protein intake
Supports muscle and metabolism.

4. Avoiding long fasting windows
Destroys testosterone.

5. Using walking for belly fat reduction
Walking + consistent meals = visceral fat reduction.

THE GREATEST MISUNDERSTANDING BETWEEN MEN AND WOMEN

Women think:
"Why can he eat whatever he wants and lose weight?"
Men think:
"Why is she working harder than me but losing slower?"
Both misunderstand biology.
Men and women have DIFFERENT metabolic rules.
Once you understand those rules, everything makes sense and no one feels "broken."

COACH'S CORNER

Look — you can't compare yourself to anybody else.
Not your spouse, not your friend, not people online.
Your biology is YOUR biology.
Women:
You are not failing.
You are not slow.

The Metabolism Reset

You are not broken.

Your hormones make you stronger, not weaker — you just need a plan that respects them.

Men:

You don't get a free pass.

Your metabolism is simpler, but you can destroy it just as fast with bad habits.

You need structure too.

Everybody:

This reset works for YOU — the real you, the hormonal you, the biological you — because it honors how your body was designed.

You're not fighting your hormones anymore.

You're working with them.

This is where real transformation happens.

CHAPTER 19

THE PSYCHOLOGY OF LONG-TERM SUCCESS

Building the Mindset, Identity, and Emotional Discipline Needed to Stay Consistent for Life — Without Dieting, Guilt, or Perfectionism

You can reset your metabolism.

You can fix your hormones.

You can heal digestion.

You can lose weight.

You can feel better than you've ever felt in your life.

But if your mindset stays rooted in diet culture — if you don't change your relationship with food, your identity, and your internal dialogue — you'll eventually fall back into the patterns that damaged your metabolism in the first place.

The truth is simple:

Long-term success is not about what you eat.

It's about how you THINK.

This chapter will teach you how to build the mental foundation required for lifelong success:

- sustainable discipline
- emotional detachment
- identity transformation
- self-trust
- confidence
- lifestyle integration
- freedom from guilt

Let's rebuild the mental side of your metabolism.

THE IDENTITY SHIFT: WHO YOU BECOME MATTERS MORE THAN WHAT YOU DO

Most people try to change their habits without changing their identity.

The Metabolism Reset

That never works.

If you still see yourself as:

- a dieter
- someone who always falls off
- someone who "loves junk food too much"
- someone who is inconsistent
- someone with no willpower
- someone who has always struggled with weight
- someone who "messes up" easily

…then no matter how well the Metabolism Reset works, your OLD identity will eventually pull you back.

Identity drives behavior.
Behavior drives results.

The goal is to shift your identity from:

"I'm trying to lose weight." → to → "I'm someone who takes care of my body."

"I'm bad around food." → to → "I trust my hunger and I fuel myself."

"I don't have discipline." → to → "I honor my commitments to myself."

"I always start over." → to → "This is just who I am now."

When your identity changes, your habits become automatic — not forced.

THE TRUTH ABOUT DISCIPLINE (YOU DON'T NEED MORE OF IT)

People think success is about discipline.

It's not.

Discipline is unreliable because it's based on:

- mood
- energy
- stress

- emotions
- environment
- motivation

Motivation fades.

Willpower runs out.

What truly creates long-term success is:

Systems.

Routine.

Structure.

Environment.

Identity.

When you rely on discipline, you burn out.

When you rely on systems, you succeed effortlessly.

The Metabolism Reset trains your system — not your discipline.

HOW TO BREAK THE "ALL-OR-NOTHING" MINDSET FOREVER

The #1 psychological killer of fat loss is all-or-nothing thinking.

It sounds like:

"I messed up, so the whole day is ruined."

"I ate one bad thing… might as well binge now."

"I'll restart Monday."

"I failed again."

This mindset DESTROYS consistency.

To break it, adopt this simple principle:

Every decision is its own decision.

Not connected to the last one.

Not tied to the next one.

Not part of a pattern unless you decide it is.

If you eat something outside the plan:

The Metabolism Reset

You didn't "fail."

You didn't "break" anything.

You didn't ruin your progress.

You just made one decision.

The next one is entirely yours.

This is emotional maturity around food.

THE POWER OF NEUTRALITY (STOP LABELING FOOD AS GOOD OR BAD)

Food is not moral.

- Eating cake doesn't make you bad.
- Eating broccoli doesn't make you good.
- Eating too much doesn't mean you failed.
- Eating less doesn't mean you succeeded.

Food is fuel.

Food is information.

Food is biology.

When you remove the emotional charge around food, you remove the guilt that triggers overeating.

Neutrality is freedom.

When food becomes neutral, you:
- stop bingeing
- stop obsessing
- stop restricting
- stop fearing hunger
- stop punishing yourself

That neutrality is necessary for lifelong metabolic health.

SELF-TRUST: THE REAL REASON MOST PEOPLE FAIL

Dieting destroys self-trust.

Every time you:

- start a new diet
- quit
- binge
- starve
- restart
- fall off
- punish yourself
- reset
- repeat

…you erode your internal trust in YOU.

And without self-trust:

- you don't believe in your ability to change
- you sabotage yourself
- you fear food
- you underestimate your strength
- you stop following through

The Metabolism Reset rebuilds self-trust because it shows you:

- you CAN eat consistently
- you CAN trust your hunger
- you CAN follow a plan
- you CAN stop starving
- you CAN make progress
- your body WILL respond

Each day you stay consistent, you regain another piece of self-trust.

EMOTIONAL REGULATION: STOP USING FOOD TO SOFTEN LIFE

Food becomes a coping mechanism when:

- life feels overwhelming
- you're lonely

- you're stressed
- you feel unseen
- you feel unappreciated
- you're exhausted
- you're anxious

People eat not because of hunger, but because they want relief.

The Reset stabilizes hormones, which reduces emotional hunger — but the mental pattern may still exist.

To break emotional eating long-term, ask yourself:

"What am I actually feeling right now?"

"What do I really need?"

99% of the time, the real need is:

- rest
- connection
- relief
- comfort
- validation
- calm
- space

Not food.

This is emotional intelligence — and it's a skill, not something you're born with.

SABOTAGE: WHY PEOPLE RUIN THEIR OWN PROGRESS

Self-sabotage happens when:

- your identity hasn't caught up to your progress
- you don't truly believe you can succeed long-term
- you're afraid of change
- success feels unfamiliar

- comfort feels safer than transformation

People don't sabotage because they're weak.

They sabotage because the NEW version of themselves feels uncomfortable.

The key to beating sabotage is:

Normalize success.

Expect success.

Choose success as your identity.

When success becomes familiar, sabotage disappears.

LONG-TERM CONSISTENCY: THE "GOOD ENOUGH RULE"

Perfection is the enemy of progress.

The "Good Enough Rule" states:

If you follow the plan 80–90% of the time, you will ALWAYS stay on track.

Not 100%.

Not perfection.

Not flawless performance.

Just consistent, stable effort.

Good enough always beats perfect.

Good enough is sustainable.

Good enough creates long-term results.

Good enough is what real life requires.

THE 5 PILLARS OF A LIFELONG METABOLIC MINDSET

If you want to maintain your results forever, build these habits into your identity:

Pillar 1: Predictability

Meals, sleep, hydration, movement.

The Metabolism Reset

Consistency = stability.

Pillar 2: Flexibility

Life happens.

Your metabolism is not fragile.

You recover easily because you know how.

Pillar 3: Neutrality

Food is not emotional.

It is just fuel.

Pillar 4: Ownership

Your success is yours.

Your choices are yours.

Your comeback is yours.

Pillar 5: Identity

You become the type of person who:

- eats consistently
- listens to hunger
- respects their body
- chooses long-term health
- doesn't quit

This identity will carry you through any challenge.

COACH'S CORNER

Listen — you can learn every strategy in this book.

You can memorize every hormone.

You can understand metabolism like a scientist.

But if your mind still thinks like a dieter…

you'll stay stuck in diet mentality.

You're not a dieter anymore.
You're not someone trying to lose weight.
You're not someone who "needs to get back on track."
You are becoming someone who eats with intention.
You are becoming someone who honors their biology.
You are becoming someone who takes care of their body.
You are becoming someone who doesn't rely on willpower
— but on SYSTEMS.
You are becoming someone who succeeds because success
is who you ARE now.
This isn't just a weight-loss program.
This is an identity shift.
This is a mindset transformation.
This is freedom.
Welcome to the life you were supposed to live.

CHAPTER 20

HOW TO BUILD A METABOLISM-FRIENDLY KITCHEN

The Foods, Tools, and Systems You Need to Keep Your Hormones Stable, Your Meals Consistent, and Your Life Stress-Free

Most people fail at nutrition not because they lack discipline…

but because their environment is built for failure.

If your kitchen is full of:

- processed snacks
- convenience foods
- sugary treats
- empty-calorie carbs
- oil-heavy meals
- "emergency" junk
- high-reward, low-nutrition items

…then your hormones don't stand a chance.

If you want to live in a high-metabolism body, you have to create a high-metabolism environment.

This chapter teaches you:

- what foods to keep
- what foods to avoid
- how to grocery shop
- how to meal prep without stress
- how to stock snacks correctly
- what tools make healthy eating easy
- how to set up your kitchen for automatic success

Let's build the environment that supports the life you want.

THE METABOLISM-FRIENDLY KITCHEN: THE RULE OF THREE

There are three core categories your kitchen must always support:

1. Convenience

If healthy food isn't convenient, you won't choose it consistently.

2. Predictability

Your environment should match your eating rhythm.

3. Preparedness

You should NEVER be caught in a "there's nothing to eat" moment.

Without these three pillars, even the best plan falls apart.

With them, your success becomes automatic.

SECTION 1: THE FOODS YOU SHOULD ALWAYS HAVE STOCKED

These foods are metabolic gold — they stabilize blood sugar, improve hormonal balance, support digestion, and reduce cravings.

PROTEINS (The Foundation)

Protein is the anchor of EVERY meal.

Always have:

- Chicken breast or thighs
- Ground turkey
- Lean beef

- Grass-fed beef (optional)
- Salmon
- Tuna packets
- Shrimp
- Eggs
- Greek yogurt
- Cottage cheese
- Clean protein powder

Protein keeps metabolism high and hunger stable.

COMPLEX CARBOHYDRATES (Hormone Regulators)

Carbs are NOT the enemy — inconsistent carbs are.

Keep:

- Rice (white or brown)
- Potatoes (gold, red, sweet)
- Oats
- Quinoa
- Whole-wheat pasta
- Beans (black, pinto, navy)
- Lentils

These carbs stabilize insulin and support metabolic repair.

FRUITS (The Natural Sweetener)

Fruits:

- satisfy cravings
- stabilize blood sugar
- reduce inflammation
- provide antioxidants

Best choices:

- berries
- bananas
- apples

- oranges
- pineapple
- grapes

Always pick whole fruit, NOT juice.

VEGETABLES (The Volume Foods)

Vegetables add nutrients without overwhelming calories.
Stock:

- spinach
- broccoli
- peppers
- green beans
- carrots
- zucchini
- onions
- mixed greens
- cauliflower

Fresh or frozen — same nutritional value.

HEALTHY FATS (Hormone Support)

Fats are essential for hormone production.
Have:

- avocado
- olive oil
- nuts (almonds, cashews, walnuts)
- seeds
- nut butters

Use them wisely — fats are dense, but powerful.

SECTION 2: THE FOODS YOU SHOULD REMOVE OR LIMIT

These foods sabotage metabolism because they trigger:

- hunger spikes
- cravings
- blood sugar crashes
- inflammation
- hormonal imbalance
- binge urges

This doesn't mean you "can never eat them."

It means:

They shouldn't live in your home.

If you want a treat, go get it — don't keep it stocked.

Remove or drastically limit:

- sugary cereals
- pastries
- candy
- chips
- fried foods
- frozen dinners
- processed meats
- soda
- energy drinks
- "healthy-looking" snacks with junk ingredients
- protein bars loaded with sugar alcohols

Your kitchen shouldn't tempt you — it should support you.

SECTION 3: GROCERY SHOPPING FOR A HIGH METABOLISM

Here is the simplest rule:

Shop the perimeter of the store.

That's where whole foods live.

The middle aisles contain:

- boxed foods
- processed snacks

- packaged sugar
- ultra-processed "health foods"

Your cart should look like:

- 80% whole foods
- 20% optional extras

Let's break grocery shopping down into categories.

THE 10-MINUTE GROCERY SHOPPING SYSTEM

A fast, stress-free system:

Category 1: Protein (Choose 3–5)
Examples:

- chicken
- turkey
- eggs
- yogurt
- salmon

Category 2: Carbs (Choose 2–3)

- potatoes
- rice
- oats
- fruit

Category 3: Vegetables (Choose 3–4)

- greens
- broccoli
- peppers
- mixed veggies

Category 4: Snacks (Choose 2)

Whole-food snacks ONLY:

- nuts
- fruit
- clean jerky
- veggies + hummus

Category 5: Extras (Choose 1)

- coffee
- seasoning
- a treat for later (not for stocking)

This keeps your kitchen ready without overbuying or stressing.

SECTION 4: SIMPLE MEAL PREP (WITHOUT FEELING LIKE A CHEF)

Meal prep should NOT:

- take hours
- require fancy recipes
- make you hate Sundays
- turn you into a full-time cook

Meal prep should be EASY.

Here is the 20-minute meal prep formula.

STEP 1: Cook 1 protein in bulk

Choose:

- chicken
- turkey
- beef
- salmon

Cook enough for 3–4 days.

STEP 2: Prepare 1–2 carb bases

Examples:

- rice
- potatoes
- quinoa

Meals become mix-and-match.

STEP 3: Chop or steam vegetables
Or buy pre-washed, pre-cut bags.
No shame — convenience beats perfection.

STEP 4: Portion a few snacks
Such as:

- nuts
- yogurt
- fruit
- veggies

When snacks are prepped, you never skip your rhythm.

STEP 5: Store everything visibly
People eat what they SEE.
Your fridge should make your success obvious.

SECTION 5: SNACK SYSTEMS THAT SUPPORT HORMONES

Snacks during the Reset are strategic — they keep:

- blood sugar stable
- cortisol low
- ghrelin rhythm consistent

Your snacks should include:

- protein
- fruit
- whole-food carbs

- healthy fats (light amounts)

Here are winning combinations:

- Greek yogurt + berries
- nuts + apple
- turkey slices + grapes
- cottage cheese + pineapple
- protein shake + banana

These snacks are metabolically stable and reduce cravings.

SECTION 6: KITCHEN TOOLS THAT MAKE THIS LIFESTYLE EASY

You don't need fancy gadgets — just tools that reduce decision-making and save time.

1. Air Fryer
Fast, easy, perfect for chicken, potatoes, veggies.

2. Instant Pot or Slow Cooker
Great for bulk proteins without effort.

3. Rice Cooker
Set it and forget it.

4. Glass Meal Containers
Portion food and SEE your meals clearly.

5. Water Bottle (Big Jug)
Hydration reminders = metabolic compliance.

6. Sharp Chef's Knife
Makes vegetable prep 10x faster.

7. Mini Cooler or Lunch Bag

Supports your eating rhythm away from home.

SECTION 7: THE "NO-EXCUSE" SYSTEM —
ALWAYS BE PREPARED

Here is the truth:

People don't fall off because of food.

They fall off because of lack of preparation.

Here is your "No-Excuse System."

1. Always have 2 emergency proteins on hand

- canned tuna
- hard-boiled eggs
- rotisserie chicken
- Greek yogurt
- clean jerky

2. Always have 2 emergency carbs ready

- fruit
- microwave rice
- potatoes cooked ahead

3. Always have 1 emergency fat source

- nuts
- avocado
- nut butter

4. Never let your fridge go empty

The moment your fridge empties…

your metabolism loses stability.

SECTION 8: EATING OUT — HOW TO STAY ON TRACK WITHOUT STRESS

You CAN eat out and maintain your metabolism.

Just follow these simple rules:

Rule 1: Protein First

Chicken, steak, fish — always anchor the meal.

Rule 2: Choose a Whole-Food Carb

Potatoes, rice, beans — avoid bread baskets and fried foods.

Rule 3: Add a Vegetable

Fiber improves digestion and fullness.

Rule 4: If you want dessert, share it

No guilt.

But don't keep it at home afterward.

THE REAL PURPOSE OF THE METABOLISM-FRIENDLY KITCHEN

Once you build this environment:

- you stop relying on discipline
- you stop fighting cravings
- you stop making emotional decisions
- you stop panicking about meals
- you stop sabotaging yourself

Your kitchen becomes the foundation of your success.

Nutrition becomes EASY.

Consistency becomes AUTOMATIC.

Metabolism stays HIGH.

This is lifestyle — not dieting.

Leonardo Lechuga

COACH'S CORNER

Look — you can't expect your metabolism to stay healed if your kitchen is working against you.

Your environment matters.

What you buy matters.

What you keep matters.

Don't make this harder than it has to be.

Stock the right foods.

Prep the simple meals.

Keep snacks ready.

Set yourself up to win.

You already did the hard part — you healed your metabolism.

Now protect that investment.

Build a kitchen that supports the life you're creating.

Your goals should be easier because of your environment — not harder.

This is how you stay consistent for LIFE.

CHAPTER 21

RECIPES & MEAL IDEAS FOR A HIGH-METABOLISM LIFESTYLE

Simple, Whole-Food Meals You Can Make Fast — No Complicated Cooking, No Diet Food, Just Real Fuel for a Real Body

Let's be honest — most people don't stick to healthy eating because they think:

- it's too time-consuming
- it's too expensive
- it's too complicated
- it requires cooking skills
- it requires fancy ingredients

Not here.

Your system is built for real people with real lives. These recipes require:

- NO professional cooking experience
- NO gourmet skills
- MINIMAL prep
- AFFORDABLE ingredients
- FAST cook times

Every recipe follows the same metabolic formula:

Protein anchor

Whole-food carbs

Vegetables or fruit

Healthy fats (optional, light)

This structure keeps hormones stable, hunger predictable, and energy high.

Let's break the meals down by category.

Leonardo Lechuga

SECTION 1: METABOLISM-BOOSTING BREAKFASTS

Breakfast is not optional in your system.

It stabilizes hormones, regulates hunger cues, and prevents late-day cravings.

Here are breakfast options that take 5 minutes or less.

1. High-Protein Scramble (5 Minutes)

Ingredients:

- 2–3 eggs
- Handful of spinach
- 2–3 tbsp diced onion or peppers
- Salt + pepper

Directions:

Scramble everything in a pan. Done.

Why it works:

Eggs stabilize hunger and improve fat burning all day.

2. Greek Yogurt Parfait

Ingredients:

- 1 cup Greek yogurt
- ½ cup berries
- 1 tbsp nuts or seeds

Directions:

Layer and enjoy.

Why it works:

Protein + fiber = balanced blood sugar.

3. Banana Protein Shake

Ingredients:

- 1 banana
- 1 scoop protein powder

- Ice + water

Directions:

Blend.

Why it works:

Fast, portable, high protein.

4. Oatmeal Power Bowl

Ingredients:

- ½ cup oats
- 1 scoop protein stirred in AFTER cooking
- Berries + cinnamon

Why it works:

Slow-digesting carbs stabilize insulin.

5. Turkey Breakfast Wrap

Ingredients:

- 1 whole wheat or low-carb wrap
- Sliced turkey
- Egg
- Spinach

Why it works:

Balanced, quick, and portable.

SECTION 2: SNACKS TO KEEP YOUR HORMONES STABLE

Your method FEEDS the metabolism.

These snacks stop crashes, cravings, and cortisol spikes.

Use these between meals every 2–3 hours.

1. Apple + Almonds

Protein + fiber + natural sugar = steady energy.

2. Turkey Slices + Grapes

Sweeter fruit reduces cravings while turkey anchors blood sugar.

3. Hard-Boiled Eggs

Simple, cheap, high-protein.

4. Cottage Cheese + Pineapple

Digestive enzymes + protein.

5. Protein Shake

For busy days or travel.

6. Veggies + Hummus

Crunchy, satisfying, nutrient-dense.

7. Banana + Peanut Butter (Light!)

Use only 1 tbsp for stable hormones.

SECTION 3: SIMPLE LUNCHES (10 MINUTES OR LESS)

Lunch needs to be predictable, balanced, and EASY.

1. Chicken + Rice + Veggies Bowl

Ingredients:

- Pre-cooked chicken
- Microwave rice
- Steamed veggies

Directions:

Assemble, season with salt or pepper.

Why it works:

Minimal thinking. Maximum balance.

2. Steak Salad Power Bowl

Ingredients:

- Leftover steak or rotisserie chicken
- Mixed greens
- Tomato
- Olive oil + balsamic

Why it works:

Protein + fiber = consistent energy.

3. Turkey Chili (Bulk Prep)

Ingredients:

- Ground turkey
- Beans
- Tomato sauce
- Onion
- Chili powder

Make once, eat for 3–4 meals.

4. Tuna & Avocado Bowl

Ingredients:

- Canned tuna
- ½ avocado
- Lemon juice
- Salt + pepper

Why it works:

High protein, no cooking, anti-inflammatory.

5. Stir Fry Meal

Ingredients:

- Frozen stir fry veggie mix
- Chicken or shrimp
- Soy sauce or coconut aminos

Leonardo Lechuga

Cooks in 7 minutes.

SECTION 4: DINNERS THAT SUPPORT FAT LOSS

Dinner doesn't need to be heavy.
It needs to be whole food based and satisfying.

1. Air-Fryer Chicken Thighs + Potatoes
Season thighs with garlic + paprika.
Air fry 20 minutes.
Add roasted potato wedges.

2. Salmon + Asparagus
Oven: 400° for 12–15 minutes.
Simple, fast, omega-3 rich.

3. Ground Turkey Meatballs + Rice
Bake or air fry.
Serve with rice or potatoes.

4. Beef + Broccoli
Sauté thin-sliced beef with broccoli.
Add low-sodium soy sauce.

5. Baked Potato + Chicken + Salsa
Cheap and incredibly filling.
Perfect for stable blood sugar.

6. Big Dinner Salad
Add: chicken, eggs, avocado, veggies.
Skip heavy dressings.

SECTION 5: FAMILY-FRIENDLY MEALS
Because your plan works in real households.

1. Whole-Wheat Pasta + Turkey Meat Sauce
Family gets pasta.
You get a stable, whole-food meal.

2. Sheet Pan Chicken Fajitas
Chicken + peppers + onions.
Serve with rice or tortillas.

3. Slow Cooker Chicken Stew
Throw ingredients in pot.
Come back to dinner.

4. Homemade Flatbread Pizza
Whole-wheat flatbread
Tomato sauce
Chicken or turkey
Vegetables
A MUCH healthier pizza that keeps hormones stable.

SECTION 6: 10-MINUTE MEALS FOR BUSY DAYS
These are "I don't feel like cooking" meals that STILL
support your metabolism.

1. Tuna Pack + Fruit + Nuts
Done in 30 seconds.

2. Avocado Toast + Eggs
Simple, balanced.

3. Rotisserie Chicken Plate

Chicken + microwave veggies + fruit.

4. Yogurt Bowl Dinner

Greek yogurt

Fruit

Nuts

Cinnamon

Perfect for late nights.

5. Breakfast for Dinner

Eggs + potatoes + fruit.

SECTION 7: FLAVOR WITHOUT SABOTAGING METABOLISM

Seasonings are your friend.

Here are metabolism-safe flavors:

- garlic
- onion powder
- paprika
- cumin
- chili powder
- lemon pepper
- Italian seasoning
- salt & pepper

Avoid heavy sauces like:

- ranch
- creamy dressings
- sugary BBQ
- Alfredo sauce
- mayo-heavy spreads

They add inflammation and unnecessary calories.

Use instead:

- salsa
- mustard
- hot sauce
- balsamic vinegar
- olive oil (light)

Real flavor. Real results.

SECTION 8: MEALS TO BREAK CRAVINGS FAST

Cravings mean one of three things:

- blood sugar instability
- low protein
- high cortisol

These meals fix that FAST.

1. Chicken + Sweet Potato

Natural sweetness + stable protein.

2. Oatmeal + Protein Powder + Berries

Great for evening cravings.

3. Eggs + Fruit

Quick hunger reset.

4. Greek Yogurt + Frozen Grapes

Tastes like dessert — fuels like a meal.

5. Cottage Cheese + Cinnamon + Honey (1 tsp)

Warm, comforting, low glycemic.

SECTION 9: TRAVEL-FRIENDLY MEALS

No fridge? No microwave? No problem.

Travel-safe staples:

- tuna pouches
- nuts
- apples
- bananas
- beef sticks (clean ingredients)
- protein shakes
- instant oats packets

Use these to maintain your eating rhythm anywhere.

SECTION 10: PUTTING IT ALL TOGETHER — SAMPLE MEAL DAYS

Here are sample days for structure.

Day Example: High-Metabolism Flow
7:00 AM — Breakfast:
Eggs + potatoes + fruit
9:30 AM — Snack:
Greek yogurt + berries
12:00 PM — Lunch:
Chicken + rice + broccoli
2:30 PM — Snack:
Fruit + nuts
5:00 PM — Dinner:
Salmon + asparagus
7:30 PM — Snack:
Protein shake (optional)
Clean. Simple. Hormone-friendly.

Day Example: Busy Lifestyle Flow
8:00 AM: Protein shake
10:00 AM: Banana + nuts

The Metabolism Reset

12:30 PM: Rotisserie chicken + veggies

3:00 PM: Cottage cheese + fruit

6:00 PM: Beef & broccoli

8:00 PM: Yogurt bowl

Effortless — but metabolically powerful.

COACH'S CORNER

Stop overthinking this.

Stop acting like you need a cookbook or a chef.

You don't need 50 ingredients.

You don't need complicated meals.

You don't need "diet food."

You need REAL food.

You need EASY food.

You need CONSISTENT food.

You need food that supports your hormones — not sabotages them.

Use these meals.

Mix them up.

Keep it simple.

Keep it whole.

Keep it balanced.

This lifestyle is supposed to feel EASY.

And these meals make it easy.

Eat like this — and your metabolism will stay on fire.

CHAPTER 22

TROUBLESHOOTING

Plateaus, Hunger Problems, Cravings, Digestion Issues, and the Most Common Metabolism Reset Mistakes — Fixed.

Even when people follow the plan well, real life brings challenges.

- Hunger feels off
- Cravings hit
- Fat loss slows
- Digestion gets weird
- Energy fluctuates
- Weight plateaus
- Stress spikes
- Sleep gets disrupted
- Schedule gets chaotic

This chapter is the ultimate guide to diagnosing the problem and fixing it — WITHOUT quitting, panicking, starving, or restarting from scratch.

Let's break down every issue you might run into and exactly what to do about it.

SECTION 1: PLATEAUS — WHY THEY HAPPEN & HOW TO BREAK THEM

Let's get this straight:

A plateau is not failure.

A plateau is communication.

Your metabolism is saying:

- "Something needs adjusting."
- "Stress is high."
- "Sleep is low."
- "Meals are inconsistent."

- "Hydration is off."
- "Hormones need recalibration."

Common Causes of Plateaus

1. Inconsistent meal timing

Skipping meals or going too long without eating disrupts ghrelin + leptin.

2. Not eating enough protein

Protein drives metabolism.

3. Not drinking enough water

Dehydration slows digestion and increases water retention.

4. Stress or cortisol spikes

High stress stops fat loss instantly.

5. Lack of movement

Walking accelerates fat loss — not movement = slower results.

6. Too much high-intensity exercise

Raises cortisol → stalls results.

7. Poor sleep

Fat loss practically shuts off with sleep disturbances.

How to Break a Plateau (The Plateau Protocol)

Do this for 72 hours:

Step 1: Eat every 2 hours again

Return to a mini-reset to stabilize hormones.

Step 2: Increase protein by 20–30g per day

Protein increases the thermic effect of food.

Step 3: Add 3,000–5,000 extra steps per day

Walking burns fat without raising cortisol.

Step 4: Reduce high-intensity workouts

Switch to strength training + walking for a few days.

Step 5: Increase water intake

Eliminate water retention + improve digestion.

Step 6: Prioritize sleep (non-negotiable)

Aim for 7–9 hours.

Plateau → broken.

SECTION 2: HUNGER FEELS TOO LOW — WHAT IT MEANS & WHAT TO DO

Low hunger is NOT a badge of honor.

It's a sign that hormones are adapting — or misfiring.

Common Causes of Low Hunger

You're still early in the reset

Ghrelin takes 10–14 days to regulate.

You're eating too much fat or heavy foods

Fat digests slowly → slows hunger return.

Cortisol is high

Stress kills appetite.

Sleep is low

Poor sleep lowers hunger signals.

You're not drinking enough water

Dehydration mimics low hunger.

You're eating too few carbs

Your body is conserving energy.

How to Fix Low Hunger

1. Eat lighter meals for 24 hours

Switch to:

- fruit
- yogurt
- eggs
- lean proteins

This speeds up digestion.

2. Increase hydration

Water triggers digestive movement → hunger returns.

3. Add 1–2 pieces of fruit per day

Fruit restores carbohydrate balance.

4. Walk after meals

Walking speeds up gastric emptying.

5. Check your sleep

If sleep is off → hunger will be off.

6. Reduce stress

Breathing exercises, light movement, quiet time.

Hunger will return — reliably — once the underlying cause is fixed.

SECTION 3: HUNGER FEELS TOO HIGH — WHAT IT MEANS & WHAT TO DO

If hunger feels "too strong," it's often a GOOD sign.

It means:

- metabolism is speeding up
- ghrelin cycles are syncing
- fat mobilization is active

But excess hunger can also mean something is off.

Common Causes of Excess Hunger

Eating too little protein

Protein keeps hunger stable.

Too much high-intensity exercise

Burns glycogen → spikes hunger.

Not enough whole-food carbs

Your body starts demanding energy.

Skipping meals

Destroys hunger rhythm.

High cortisol

Stress increases hunger.

How to Fix Excess Hunger

Step 1: Add an extra ounce or two of protein to your meals

Or add a protein snack mid-morning or mid-afternoon.

Step 2: Add more carbs (potatoes, rice, fruit)

Your metabolism is speeding up — feed it.

Step 3: Reduce high-intensity workouts for a few days

Lower cortisol → lower hunger.

Step 4: Make sure meals aren't too small

Your body is telling you it needs more fuel.

Step 5: Drink more water

Thirst often feels like hunger.

Step 6: Stick to whole foods only

Processed foods cause rebound hunger.

When metabolism revs up, hunger goes up — this is NORMAL.

SECTION 4: CRAVINGS — WHY THEY HAPPEN & HOW TO STOP THEM FAST

Cravings are not weakness.

They are hormonal messages.

Types of Cravings & What They Mean

Sugar cravings

Blood sugar crash

Low carbs

High cortisol

Dehydration

Carb cravings

Your body needs fuel — especially during PMS in women.

Chocolate cravings

The Metabolism Reset

Low magnesium

Low serotonin

Salt cravings

Dehydration

Low electrolytes

Craving Killers (Fast Fixes)

If you're craving sugar:

 Eat a piece of fruit

It satisfies cravings WITHOUT spiking insulin.

If you're craving carbs:

 Eat a potato or rice with protein

Stabilizes blood sugar.

If you're craving chocolate:

 Try dark chocolate (1–2 pieces) + nuts

Stops cravings without binging.

If you're craving salt:

 Drink a glass of water + electrolytes

If you're craving everything:

 Eat a full meal

You're under-fueled.

SECTION 5: DIGESTION ISSUES — BLOATING, CONSTIPATION, OR GAS

Digestion is directly tied to metabolism.

If digestion slows, metabolism slows.

Common Causes of Digestive Issues

Not enough water

Not enough vegetables

Too much fat

Not enough movement

Hormonal shifts
Eating too fast
Stress

Fixes for Bloating
Walk after meals (10–15 minutes)
Reduces gas + speeds digestion.
Reduce heavy fats for 24 hours
Let your stomach reset.
Drink warm water or peppermint tea
Relaxes digestive muscles.
Avoid carbonated drinks
Traps gas.

Fixes for Constipation
Increase water
Add fruit (especially kiwi, pears, berries)
Add vegetables
Add magnesium at night (supplement optional)
Add walking
Reduce dairy for 24 hours

Fixes for Gas
Cook vegetables instead of eating raw
Reduce beans temporarily
Eat slowly
Limit chewing gum
Avoid artificial sweeteners

SECTION 6: ENERGY CRASHES — WHAT THEY MEAN

If energy is crashing, one of these is happening:

- you're under-eating
- meals are inconsistent
- carbs are too low
- sleep is off
- hydration is low
- cortisol is high

Fix Energy Crashes Fast
Eat a balanced snack: protein + carbs
Drink water
Walk for 5–10 minutes
Eat more whole-food carbs
Reduce caffeine for 24 hours
Prioritize sleep that night
Energy is the first sign of hormonal stability.

SECTION 7: THE MOST COMMON MISTAKES PEOPLE MAKE (AND HOW TO FIX THEM)
Let's be honest — most mistakes are simple.
Mistake #1: Not eating every 2–3 hours
Fix: Set timers.

Mistake #2: Eating too much fat
Fix: Keep fats light — fats slow digestion.

Mistake #3: Skipping breakfast
Fix: Eat within 60 minutes of waking.

Mistake #4: Not drinking enough water
Fix: 60–100 oz per day depending on body size.

Mistake #5: High-intensity workouts too often

Fix: Walk more, lift weights intentionally.

Mistake #6: Eating too little protein
Fix: Aim for 20–30g per meal.

Mistake #7: Not preparing snacks ahead
Fix: Keep emergency snacks ready ALWAYS.

Mistake #8: Keeping junk food in the house
Fix: If it's not there, you won't eat it.

Mistake #9: Treating this like a diet
Fix: This is metabolic repair — not restriction.

Mistake #10: Panicking at small weight fluctuations
Fix: Weight fluctuates — the process is consistent.

SECTION 8: WHEN TO TIGHTEN UP VS WHEN TO RELAX

Tighten up when:
- hunger is inconsistent
- cravings are intense
- stress is high
- sleep is poor
- meals are irregular
- digestion feels off
- you're traveling

Return to the mini-reset (every 2 hours).

Relax when:
- hunger is predictable
- hormones feel stable

- meals are consistent
- digestion is good
- fat loss is steady
- stress is low

This is metabolic freedom.

COACH'S CORNER

Look — troubleshooting ain't punishment.

It's not starting over.

It's not failing.

It's how you LEARN your body.

Your metabolism talks to you every day.

Hunger tells you something.

Cravings tell you something.

Digestion tells you something.

Energy tells you something.

Plateaus tell you something.

Nothing here is random.

Nothing is broken.

Nothing is your fault.

You're not guessing anymore — you've got the blueprint.

You know how to fix ANY issue quickly.

And once you can troubleshoot yourself?

You become unstoppable.

This is how you turn a temporary reset into a lifelong lifestyle.

CHAPTER 23

THE ATHLETE'S GUIDE TO THE METABOLISM RESET

How Fighters, Martial Artists, and High-Performance Athletes Can Reset Their Metabolism Without Losing Strength, Energy, or Performance

Let's get one thing straight:

Athletes cannot follow the same rules as the general population.

Your engine runs hotter.

Your hormonal needs are different.

Your caloric output is higher.

And under-eating will destroy your performance faster than anything.

This chapter is for the fighters, the grapplers, the kickboxers, the boxers, the MMA athletes, the competitors, and the hard-training hobbyists who push their bodies 4–6 days a week.

Your needs are different — and if you don't respect that, you will:

- overtrain
- burn out
- lose strength
- flatten your hormones
- ruin recovery
- crash during training
- hit plateaus
- lose muscle
- or worse — get injured

The Metabolism Reset WORKS for athletes — but the rules must be applied with intention and knowledge.

Let's dive in.

SECTION 1: ATHLETES RUN DIFFERENT HORMONAL SYSTEMS

High-intensity training affects:

- cortisol
- insulin
- adrenaline
- testosterone
- growth hormone
- thyroid hormones
- ghrelin (hunger)
- leptin (satiety)

When you train hard, your body:

- burns through glycogen
- tears muscle fibers
- increases inflammation
- activates stress hormones
- accelerates metabolic turnover

Which means:

You MUST eat more.

You MUST eat more frequently.

You CANNOT skip meals.

You CANNOT rely on discipline alone.

The average person's metabolism can be reset with structure.

The athlete's metabolism needs structure, fuel, and precision timing.

SECTION 2: THE BIGGEST MISTAKES ATHLETES MAKE (THAT DESTROY METABOLISM)

Let's call this out with tough love:

Mistake #1: Training hard while under-eating

Leonardo Lechuga

You cannot run a Ferrari on fumes.

Yet athletes do it all the time.

Signs of under-eating:

- crash in sparring rounds
- getting tired faster than usual
- shaky hands
- headaches
- irritability
- decreased strength
- trouble making decisions while rolling
- plateau in progress
- injuries
- slow recovery

Under-eating is the fastest way to destroy an athlete's performance.

Mistake #2: Training fasted

Athletes should NEVER train without fuel.

Training fasted:

- raises cortisol
- increases muscle breakdown
- decreases speed
- lowers reaction time
- increases injury risk

It's not "discipline" — it's sabotage.

Mistake #3: Not eating enough carbs

Carbs = ENERGY.

When athletes cut carbs:

- sparring suffers
- conditioning crashes
- endurance drops

- testosterone drops
- recovery slows

Your sport is explosive — it requires glucose.

Mistake #4: Ignoring recovery nutrition
If you don't eat the right way after training:

- lactic acid stays elevated
- muscle tears heal slower
- inflammation stays high
- glycogen stays depleted

Recovery nutrition is mandatory.

Mistake #5: Thinking the Metabolism Reset is a weight-cutting program
No — this is a healing program.
Weight cutting is a DIFFERENT strategy done SHORT-TERM for competition.
The Reset is about restoring hormonal power.

SECTION 3: HOW THE METABOLISM RESET WORKS FOR ATHLETES
The rules are similar to the standard reset, but with key modifications.
Eat every 2–3 hours
Athletes burn through energy faster.
Increase total calories
This is a MUST.
Add more whole-food carbs
Rice, potatoes, fruit — these are your allies.
Increase protein intake
You need muscle repair every single day.
Hydrate at a higher standard

Electrolytes are mandatory.

Maintain consistent meal timing

Your hormones rely on it.

Avoid long fasting windows

Fasting destroys athletic performance.

Reduce high-intensity training during the first 7–10 days if needed

Not required for everyone — but important to warn.

SECTION 4: WHAT ATHLETES SHOULD EXPECT DURING THE RESET

Let's be honest — the first 1–2 weeks might feel weird:

- hunger might be off
- energy might fluctuate
- body might feel heavier at first
- muscles may feel fuller
- water retention may increase temporarily
- conditioning may dip slightly in week 1

Why?

Because your body is rebalancing its hormones.

Then suddenly — around week 2–3 — athletes feel:

- more energy
- more endurance
- better sleep
- faster reaction time
- increased strength
- deeper recovery
- better cardio
- less inflammation

That's what happens when the metabolism stabilizes.

SECTION 5: HOW MUCH SHOULD ATHLETES EAT? (GUIDELINES)

Athletes should NOT eat like the general public.

This is a simple formula:

Protein Requirement

Aim for:

0.8–1 gram of protein per pound of bodyweight

Example:

A 180 lb athlete needs 150–180g of protein daily.

Carbohydrate Requirement

This is the biggest difference.

Athletes need:

1.5–3 grams of carbs per pound of bodyweight (depending on training intensity)

Carbs MUST be:

- rice
- potatoes
- oats
- beans
- fruit

NOT:

- bread
- pasta
- cereal
- processed snacks
- sugary drinks

Fats

Light intake:

- avocado
- olive oil

Leonardo Lechuga

- nuts
- seeds

Avoid heavy fats pre-training — they slow digestion and energy.

SECTION 6: HOW ATHLETES SHOULD TIME THEIR FOOD

This is the key to maximizing performance.

PRE-TRAINING MEAL (60–90 minutes before)

Eat:

- protein + complex carbs
- NO heavy fats
- NO junk
- NO high fiber (slows digestion)

Examples:

- chicken + rice
- eggs + potatoes
- yogurt + fruit
- tuna + sweet potato

This meal fuels technique, sparring, and endurance.

IMMEDIATE POST-TRAINING MEAL (0–30 minutes after)

This meal MUST contain:

Fast carbs (fruit or rice)

Replenishes glycogen.

Protein (20–30g minimum)

Repairs muscle.

Examples:

- banana + protein shake
- rice + chicken

- Greek yogurt + fruit

This meal prevents:

- muscle breakdown
- next-day soreness
- slow recovery
- cortisol spikes

SECOND POST-TRAINING MEAL (1–2 hours later)

This reinforces:

- hormone stability
- muscle repair
- inflammation reduction

Should include:

- protein
- carbs
- vegetables
- light fats

SECTION 7: HOW TO TRAIN WHILE ON THE RESET

If you're still eating consistently, you do NOT need to decrease training intensity long-term.

But for the first 7–10 days:

Jiu-Jitsu: keep rolls technical

Muay Thai/Boxing: reduce max-intensity pad rounds

Strength training: stay moderate

Conditioning circuits: reduce volume

Once hunger normalizes → performance skyrockets.

SECTION 8: SAMPLE DAY FOR A HARD-TRAINING ATHLETE

Let's create a real-life example.

Leonardo Lechuga

Morning
Breakfast:
Eggs + fruit + potatoes
Snack:
Greek yogurt + berries
Lunch
Chicken + rice + veggies
Snack:
Turkey slices + banana
Pre-training meal
Chicken + sweet potato
Post-training snack (immediate)
Protein shake + fruit
Dinner
Beef + rice + vegetables
Evening Snack
Cottage cheese + pineapple
This supports:

- intense sparring
- weightlifting
- cardio sessions
- tactical training

SECTION 9: ATHLETES WHO MAKE THESE ADJUSTMENTS GET INCREDIBLE RESULTS

Athletes often see:

- increased stamina
- faster recovery
- better rolling quality
- improved focus
- increased strength
- reduced inflammation

- improved joint health
- reduced anxiety
- stable energy
- reduced cravings
- better body composition

Because…

A fueled athlete is a dangerous athlete.

An underfed athlete is an injured athlete.

COACH'S CORNER

Look — if you're training 4–5 days a week, you don't get to eat like a regular person.

You don't get to skip breakfast.

You don't get to "forget" snacks.

You don't get to show up to Jiu-Jitsu on an empty stomach.

You don't get to pretend discipline replaces fuel.

You're an athlete.

That means you need structure, fuel, hydration, and consistency.

When you follow this reset the right way?

Your gas tank stays full.

Your recovery improves.

Your cardio gets smoother.

Your rolls get sharper.

Your kicks get cleaner.

Your reaction time tightens up.

You feel UNSTOPPABLE — because you're finally feeding your body the way an athlete should.

Fuel like a champion.

Train like a champion.

Recover like a champion.

And your performance will show it.

CHAPTER 24

THE VEGETARIAN WHOLE-FOOD RESET

How to Heal Your Metabolism on a Plant-Forward Diet Without Relying on Fake Meat, Processed Soy, or Junk Masquerading as "Healthy"

Let's be clear about something right away:

Vegetarians CAN absolutely succeed on the Metabolism Reset.

But they MUST structure their meals deliberately.

A plant-based diet does NOT automatically mean healthy.

A lot of vegetarians struggle not because of the lifestyle —

but because of the foods marketed to them:

- fake meats
- soy patties
- plant-based burgers
- ultra-processed meat substitutes
- protein bars
- sugary yogurts
- granola cereals
- seed-oil-loaded "vegan snacks"
- processed meat alternatives filled with fillers and chemicals

None of that is whole food.

None of that supports a stable metabolism.

All of that destroys hormone balance.

This chapter teaches vegetarians how to reset their metabolism using real, whole, nutrient-rich foods — not fake health products.

SECTION 1: THE BIGGEST CHALLENGES VEGETARIANS FACE

Vegetarians usually struggle with four things:

1. Too many carbs, not enough protein

Carbs are great — when balanced with protein.

Most vegetarians eat:

- pasta
- bread
- cereal
- grains
- fruit
- beans

But even the healthiest carbs don't create stable hormones by themselves.

Protein is mandatory for:

- muscle recovery
- hunger control
- metabolism
- hormone production

Without it, the Reset becomes inconsistent.

2. Relying on processed "fake meats"

Let's call this out plainly:

If your "vegetarian meat" has 25 ingredients, weird chemicals, gums, emulsifiers, seed oils, and soy isolates — it's not food. It's a science project.

These foods:

- cause inflammation
- create bloating
- disrupt hormones
- spike cravings

- destroy gut health

They have NO place in a metabolic healing program.

3. Not getting complete proteins

Animal proteins contain all essential amino acids.

Plant proteins must be paired correctly to achieve this.

Without proper pairing, vegetarians may experience:

- low energy
- slow recovery
- muscle loss
- cravings
- brain fog

All preventable with proper planning.

4. Nutrient deficiencies

Vegetarians often become deficient in:

- B12
- iron
- omega-3s
- zinc
- iodine

All of these impact metabolism and hormones.

This chapter will show how to prevent ALL of these issues.

SECTION 2: THE VEGETARIAN WHOLE-FOOD RULES

To thrive on this reset, vegetarians must follow these guidelines:

Rule #1: Whole Food Comes First

The Metabolism Reset

No fake meats.

No soy-based junk.

No filler-loaded meat substitutes.

No plant-based "nuggets," "burgers," or "sausages" with 16 paragraphs of ingredients.

Stick to REAL foods:

- lentils
- chickpeas
- beans
- quinoa
- tofu (minimally processed, organic)
- tempeh (fermented soy — MUCH healthier)
- eggs (if ovo-vegetarian)
- dairy (if lacto-vegetarian)
- nuts
- seeds
- vegetables
- fruits

Rule #2: Protein Must Be Prioritized

You MUST incorporate protein with EVERY meal and snack.

This prevents:

- cravings
- blood sugar spikes
- mood instability
- overeating
- muscle loss

Vegetarian protein sources include:

High-Protein Whole Foods:

- lentils
- chickpeas

- black beans
- kidney beans
- navy beans
- tofu (organic, non-GMO)
- tempeh
- Greek yogurt
- cottage cheese
- eggs

Protein Combinations That Create Complete Proteins:

- beans + rice
- lentils + nuts
- quinoa + beans
- oats + yogurt
- chickpeas + whole grains

Use these pairings daily.

Rule #3: Keep Carbs Whole and Intentional

Vegetarians often overeat carbs accidentally.

Carbs you SHOULD choose:

- potatoes
- sweet potatoes
- rice
- oats
- quinoa
- fruit
- vegetables
- lentils
- beans

Carbs to reduce or avoid:

- breads
- tortillas
- cereals

- granola
- pasta
- crackers
- snack foods
- fruit juices

Whole carbs = stable hormones.

Processed carbs = unstable cravings.

Rule #4: Combine Protein + Carbs Every 2–3 Hours

Vegetarians especially benefit from this because plant-based proteins digest faster.

Eating rhythm prevents:

- hunger spikes
- low energy
- grazing
- overeating
- carb overload
- blood sugar crashes

Rule #5: Avoid All Seed Oils

Vegetarian foods are often LOADED with seed oils:

- canola
- soybean
- safflower
- sunflower
- corn oil
- cottonseed oil

Seed oils cause:

- inflammation
- digestive issues
- hormone imbalance
- cravings
- bloating

Leonardo Lechuga

Use instead:

- olive oil (REAL olive oil)
- avocado oil
- coconut oil
- butter or ghee (if allowed)

SECTION 3: HOW VEGETARIANS HIT PROTEIN GOALS

Here's your biggest asset:

Protein is absolutely achievable on a vegetarian diet —
IF you structure it correctly.

Let's break it down.

Eggs (if allowed)
Perfect protein.
Support hormones.
Easy to digest.
Great for breakfast or snacks.

Greek Yogurt & Cottage Cheese
High-protein, low sugar, extremely filling.
Mix with:

- berries
- nuts
- honey (light)
- cinnamon

Lentils
One of the BEST vegetarian foods on earth.
High protein.
High fiber.
Extremely stabilizing.

The Metabolism Reset

Use in:

- soups
- stews
- salads
- bowls

Beans

Black beans, kidney beans, chickpeas — all excellent.
Pair with rice to create a complete protein.

Tofu & Tempeh

Tempeh is far superior to tofu because it is:

- fermented
- easier to digest
- nutrient-rich
- less processed

Choose organic, non-GMO, minimally processed options.

Quinoa

One of the few plant foods that is a COMPLETE protein by itself.

Use as:

- base for bowls
- side dish
- salad topper

Nuts & Seeds

Not high enough in protein alone — but fantastic as add-ons.

Great options:

- almonds
- walnuts

- pumpkin seeds
- hemp seeds
- chia seeds

SECTION 4: SAMPLE VEGETARIAN MEAL DAY

Here is a balanced, metabolism-safe, whole-food vegetarian day.

Breakfast
Greek yogurt + berries + chia seeds
or
Eggs + spinach + potatoes

Snack
Banana + almonds
or
Cottage cheese + pineapple

Lunch
Lentil + quinoa bowl
with vegetables + olive oil + salt

Snack
Hummus + vegetables
or
Fruit + nuts

Dinner
Tofu or tempeh stir fry
with rice + vegetables

Evening Snack

Protein shake (minimal-ingredient plant protein)

or

Greek yogurt

SECTION 5: PLANT-BASED PROTEIN POWDERS — WHAT TO LOOK FOR

Most plant-based protein powders are garbage.

Avoid powders with:

- artificial sweeteners
- maltodextrin
- gums and fillers
- "natural flavors"
- corn syrup solids
- seed oils
- 20+ ingredients

Choose powders with:

- pea protein
- rice protein
- hemp protein
- only 3–6 ingredients
- no artificial additives

Your protein powder should read like FOOD — not a chemistry experiment.

SECTION 6: HOW VEGETARIANS MAINTAIN METABOLIC STABILITY

To stay consistent:

Eat protein at every meal

Pair carbs with protein always

Avoid processed vegetarian foods

Eat every 2–3 hours

Hydrate

Leonardo Lechuga

Keep snacks whole-food-based
Add electrolytes
Choose REAL olive oil
Read labels

Prioritize micronutrients (B12, iron, omega-3s)
Vegetarians THRIVE when they follow these principles.

COACH'S CORNER
Look — you can do this without eating fake meat.
You can do this without living off pasta and bread.
You can do this without starving yourself or feeling weak.
You can do this without buying "healthy-looking" junk
covered in green labels and buzzwords.
You just need real food.
Whole food.
Food that your body recognizes.
Food that stabilizes your hormones, not confuses them.
Lentils, beans, quinoa, eggs, tofu, tempeh, yogurt —
that's your foundation.
Fruit, vegetables, rice, potatoes — that's your fuel.
Nuts, seeds, healthy oils — that's your support system.
You're not at a disadvantage.
You're not missing out.
Your diet is NOT a limitation.
It's just a different blueprint — and if you follow it with
intention, you will feel amazing, perform better, and heal
your metabolism just like everyone else.

CHAPTER 25

WHAT WHOLE FOODS REALLY ARE

How to Read Labels, Avoid Hidden Junk, Choose Clean Ingredients, and Build a Truly Metabolic-Friendly Diet

Let's get something absolutely clear:

Just because a package has a green leaf on it doesn't mean the food is healthy.

Just because the label says "organic" doesn't make it clean.

Just because it says "high protein" doesn't mean it's good for your metabolism.

And just because something is vegetarian, keto, gluten-free, or plant-based doesn't mean it isn't ultra-processed garbage.

Most people THINK they're eating whole foods…

But the truth?

They're eating food disguised as whole food — packed with:

- fillers
- preservatives
- gums
- stabilizers
- seed oils
- sugars
- artificial sweeteners
- lab-made "natural" flavors
- chemical thickeners
- coloring agents

Your metabolism cannot heal in that environment.

This chapter teaches you what whole foods REALLY are — and how to avoid everything pretending to be whole food.

SECTION 1: THE SIMPLE DEFINITION OF WHOLE FOOD

Let's cut the nonsense:

Leonardo Lechuga

If it grew from the earth, walked, flew, or swam — and it hasn't been altered — it's whole food.

That's it.

Examples:

- meat
- fish
- eggs
- vegetables
- fruit
- potatoes
- rice
- beans
- nuts
- seeds

If it came from the ground or from an animal — and the ingredient list is ONE WORD — it's whole food.

If it was designed in a lab with 12 chemicals?

Not whole food.

SECTION 2: THE WHOLE-FOOD PURITY STANDARD

Whole food should meet these criteria:

One ingredient

Chicken = chicken.

Rice = rice.

Peanuts = peanuts.

Olive oil = olives.

Recognizable

If your great-grandparents wouldn't recognize it, it's probably processed.

Minimally touched

Washing, cutting, freezing, grinding = fine.
Extruding, bleaching, hydrogenating, isolating = NOT fine.
Short shelf-life
Real food spoils.
Fake food lasts forever.
No additives
No gums, fillers, preservatives, "flavors," or oils.

SECTION 3: THE DANGEROUS GRAY AREA —
"HEALTHY LOOKING" FOODS THAT ARE ACTUALLY
JUNK

These foods appear healthy but destroy your metabolism.
Let's call them out:

1. Most Peanut Butter Brands
Real peanut butter ingredients should be:
peanuts + salt (optional)
That's it.
If your peanut butter contains:

- sugar
- palm oil
- vegetable oil
- "natural flavors"
- corn syrup solids
- soybean oil

Throw it away.
Those oils DESTROY metabolic health and gut function.

2. Most Protein Shakes & Powders
What companies put in protein powder today is wild:

- gums
- thickeners

- artificial sweeteners
- seed oils
- corn syrup derivatives
- heavy metals
- fillers
- dyes

A clean protein powder should have:

3–6 ingredients max

no artificial flavors

no sucralose or aspartame

no seed oils

no gums if possible

no "proprietary blends"

If you can't pronounce an ingredient, your body can't either.

3. Most Protein Bars

Protein bars are often candy bars pretending to be healthy.

Common ingredients:

- glucose syrup
- seed oils
- sugar alcohols
- glycerin
- artificial sweeteners
- "natural" flavors
- emulsifiers
- 25+ ingredients

Bars are not food.

They're processed sugar bricks.

If you need portable protein:

- nuts

- fruit
- homemade trail mix
- hard-boiled eggs
- clean jerky
- cottage cheese cups
- yogurt

Real food beats bars every time.

4. Most "Plant-Based Meats"
If your "veggie burger" has:

- 20+ ingredients
- soy isolates
- pea protein isolates
- seed oils
- emulsifiers
- gums
- stabilizers

…it's lab food.
Not whole food.

5. Salad Dressings
Most dressings contain:

- canola oil
- soybean oil
- sugar
- corn syrup
- preservatives

Even "healthy-looking" ones.
For whole-food dressing:

- olive oil
- balsamic vinegar
- lemon

- herbs
- salt

Done.

6. Granola, Cereal, and "Health Snacks"

These are dessert in disguise.

They cause blood sugar crashes, cravings, and inflammation.

Stick to:

- oats
- fruit
- nuts

Not the sugar-loaded packaged stuff.

SECTION 4: SEED OILS — THE HIDDEN METABOLIC DESTROYER

Seed oils are the biggest enemy of whole-food eating.

They include:

- canola
- soybean
- safflower
- sunflower
- corn
- cottonseed
- grapeseed

They cause:

- inflammation
- insulin resistance
- hormone disruption
- increased hunger
- cravings
- digestive issues

- sluggish metabolism

These oils are in 80–90% of packaged foods.
ALWAYS check labels.

SECTION 5: HOW TO FIND REAL OLIVE OIL

Most grocery store olive oil is fake or cut with cheaper oils.
To find REAL olive oil:
 Choose dark bottles
Light destroys purity.
 Look for "cold-pressed"
Not heat extracted.
 Look for harvest date
Not just expiration date.
 Choose brands from California, Italy, Greece, or Spain with certification.
 It should taste peppery
Real olive oil has flavor — not blandness.

SECTION 6: GOOD SALT VS BAD SALT

Salt matters more than people think.
Bad Salt:

- iodized table salt
- bleached
- anti-caking agents
- stripped of minerals

This salt actually works AGAINST hormone balance.

Good Salt:

- Himalayan pink salt
- Celtic sea salt
- Redmond Real Salt

These contain:

- magnesium
- calcium
- potassium
- trace minerals

Your hormones NEED minerals for proper function.

SECTION 7: THE CLEAN LABEL CHECKLIST
Every reader should learn this.
When looking at any food label, ask:
Does it have fewer than 5 ingredients?
Are all ingredients whole and recognizable?
Are there ANY seed oils?
Are there ANY sweeteners?
Are there ANY gums or fillers?
Does it spoil naturally?
Would my great-grandparents understand it?
If it fails these tests → it's not whole food.

SECTION 8: WHOLE FOOD EXAMPLES LIST
Here is a simple list of TRUE whole foods:
Meat
beef, chicken, turkey, lamb, fish
Eggs
one ingredient, perfect metabolically
Vegetables
spinach, broccoli, peppers, potatoes, carrots
Fruits
berries, bananas, apples, citrus, grapes
Grains
rice, oats, quinoa, barley
Legumes
beans, lentils, chickpeas, peas

Nuts & Seeds

almonds, walnuts, pumpkin seeds, chia seeds

Healthy Oils

REAL olive oil, avocado oil, coconut oil

If a food doesn't fit in one of these categories — it's probably not whole.

COACH'S CORNER

Look — don't let marketing lie to you.

Don't let companies trick you with pretty labels and buzzwords.

Most of the stuff sold as "healthy" is absolute trash.

If you want to heal your metabolism, you gotta eat REAL food.

Food with one ingredient.

Food you can recognize.

Food your body was designed to digest — not food made in some lab by people in white coats.

Real peanut butter has TWO ingredients max.

Real olive oil comes in dark bottles and tastes alive.

Real salt isn't bleached white.

Real protein doesn't come with 18 chemicals attached.

Real food doesn't need marketing — it speaks for itself.

The cleaner the ingredient list…

The cleaner your hormones.

The cleaner your metabolism.

The cleaner your results.

Keep it real — your body will thank you for it.

CHAPTER 26

REAL SUCCESS STORIES & TRUE TESTIMONIALS

Transformations From Real People Who Experienced the Metabolism Reset First-Hand

One of the most powerful ways to understand this method is to see how it has worked for real people — not theories, not guesses, not marketing claims. These are true testimonials from individuals who followed the Metabolism Reset under my guidance. Their backgrounds are different. Their goals were different. But their results came from the same principles:

stop starving, start fueling, balance hormones, trust biology.

These stories demonstrate what's possible when the body finally gets what it needs.

TESTIMONIAL 1 — The Overtrained Weightlifter Who Was Eating Only 800 Calories

Starting Weight: ~200 lbs

What She Was Doing:

- Lifting 2 hours a day
- Kickboxing private lessons
- Personal trainer restricting her to ~800 calories
- Spending $300/month on supplements
- Plateaued, exhausted, discouraged
- Publicly ready to quit altogether

This woman was doing everything "the fitness industry" tells people to do:

Lift heavy, train hard, cut calories, stack supplements, and push through exhaustion.

But her body was shutting down.

The Metabolism Reset

When I saw her frustrated social media post, I reached out. She explained:

- She wasn't losing weight
- She wasn't gaining strength
- She was exhausted every day
- She felt stuck in a permanent plateau
- Her personal trainer insisted she keep lowering calories

In our consultation, it took about 30 seconds for me to see the real issue:

She wasn't overweight — she was starving.

Her metabolism wasn't slow — it was suppressed.

Her body wasn't broken — it was under attack.

We threw out the 800-calorie starvation diet.

We threw out the unnecessary supplements.

We rebuilt her metabolism through structured whole-food meals every 2 hours.

RESULTS:

Within 3 weeks, she dropped from 200 lbs to 185 lbs — while eating more than she'd eaten in months.

She eventually reached between 160–165 lbs, stabilized there, and maintained it with ease. Her energy returned. Her strength increased. Her plateaus broke.

She didn't fail her diet.

Her diet failed her.

Once her metabolism was repaired, her body did exactly what it was supposed to do.

TESTIMONIAL 2 — The 6-Week Weight Loss Challenge Participant Who Lost Over 30 Pounds

During a gym-wide 6-week challenge, we monitored training closely and gave specific diet recommendations. One young woman was assigned to follow the Metabolism Reset exactly.

She took it seriously.

She carried a lunchbox everywhere — apples, tuna packs, whole-food snacks — eating every 2 hours without missing a beat.

She stopped starving.

She stopped skipping meals.

She stopped relying on "diet foods."

She fueled correctly and consistently.

RESULTS:

In just 6 weeks, she lost over 30 pounds.

Not water.

Not crash dieting.

Not overtraining.

Not deprivation.

Just proper fueling, hormone stabilization, and metabolic consistency.

Her discipline + the proper strategy = dramatic transformation.

TESTIMONIAL 3 — The Client Who Couldn't Lose Weight Because He Was Starving Himself

A man came to me frustrated — overweight, confused, and unable to lose a single pound despite exercising. When we reviewed his habits, we discovered the same issue I see over and over:

He was trying to lose weight by restricting calories and skipping meals.

The Metabolism Reset

He thought he needed to "eat less."

His body thought it needed to survive.

We explained that his metabolism was in full starvation mode. No food = no fat burning. The body simply refuses to release fat when it believes food is scarce.

We placed him on the structured 2-hour eating rhythm with real whole foods.

RESULTS:

His energy improved almost immediately.

His weight began dropping consistently.

His hunger normalized.

His cravings decreased.

His progress finally made sense because his biology was no longer being sabotaged.

TESTIMONIAL 4 — The Fighter Who Lost 25 Pounds in Just Over 2 Weeks

We once received a fight offer for a championship match on short notice. The fighter was already in good shape, already eating decently, and already disciplined — but we needed to drop 25 pounds in about 3 weeks.

This wasn't a case of repairing a broken metabolism.

This was a case of accelerating a healthy one.

We combined:

- The 2-hour eating structure
- Whole foods
- Zero processed junk
- A hyperhydration protocol
- Daily accountability

Within the first week he dropped small increments daily, steadily and safely.

Then — a hiccup.

Leonardo Lechuga

He went to a party, ate a huge piece of chocolate cake, and stalled for 2 days.

He came to me frustrated.

I asked him straight:

"What did you do differently?"

He confessed.

I told him the truth:

"It's fine. You didn't break the system. Stick to the plan. Your body will flush it and get right back on track."

RESULTS:

He continued the protocol and successfully dropped 25 pounds in just over 2 weeks — safely — and made championship weight.

We have used this exact method repeatedly for:

- Fighters making weight
- Athletes changing divisions
- Students preparing for tournaments

It works as a long-term metabolic repair system and a short-term competitive weight-cutting protocol.

THE COMMON THREAD IN ALL THESE REAL STORIES

Every one of these transformations had the same villain:

Starvation

Meal skipping

Calorie restriction

Overtraining

Supplement overuse

Diet myths

Metabolic confusion

And they had the same solution:

The Metabolism Reset

Eat consistently
Eat whole foods
Eat every 2 hours
Support hormones
Trust biology
Fuel instead of deprive

Their bodies weren't broken — their strategies were.

Once their metabolism was restored, their results followed naturally.

COACH'S CORNER

I didn't guess my way into these results.
I watched them happen — again and again.
When people stop starving and start fueling their body properly, the weight comes off, the energy comes back, and the plateaus disappear.
This system works because it works WITH your biology instead of against it.
These aren't theories. These are real people with real transformations.

CHAPTER 27

YOUR NEW LIFE

How to Maintain a High-Metabolism Lifestyle Forever Without Dieting, Stress, or Fear of Regaining Weight

When people finish the Metabolism Reset, they often have the same question:

"Okay… but what do I do NOW? How do I live like this without going backwards?"

This chapter is your blueprint for the rest of your life — not just the next few weeks.

The whole point of a metabolism reset is to:

- stabilize hunger
- restore hormonal balance
- repair metabolic function
- eliminate binge-restrict cycles
- create consistent energy
- teach you how your body works

Once your metabolism is healed, the goal becomes maintaining it — which is MUCH easier than most people think.

Dieting is exhausting.
Maintenance is freedom.

Let's build that freedom.

SECTION 1: THE GOLDEN LAW OF MAINTENANCE

Here is the single most important rule:

Eat consistently.
Not perfectly.
Not strictly.
Not fearfully.
Just consistently.

The Metabolism Reset

Consistency keeps:

- cortisol low
- cravings stable
- blood sugar balanced
- metabolism high
- hunger signals predictable

Your hormones LOVE routine.

SECTION 2: WHAT MAINTENANCE ACTUALLY LOOKS LIKE

Most people think maintenance is:

- strict
- stressful
- restrictive
- rigid
- boring

But true metabolic maintenance is:

- flexible
- intuitive
- predictable
- enjoyable
- sustainable
- powerful

Here's what maintenance looks like day-to-day:

Eat 3 meals and 2–3 snacks

Keep protein high

Keep carbs whole-food-based

Use fats lightly and intentionally

Drink plenty of water

Move your body daily

Sleep consistently

Don't starve

Leonardo Lechuga

Don't binge
Don't go long stretches without food
That's it.
You're not dieting anymore — you're living.

SECTION 3: HOW TO HANDLE WEEKENDS
Weekends used to be the danger zone for most people.
Not anymore.
Here's the weekend system:
Keep breakfast consistent
This anchors your hormones.
Eat every 3 hours
Even when busy, social, or relaxing.
If eating out — choose whole foods
Protein + carb + vegetable.
If having dessert — enjoy it, then move on
No guilt.
No restarting Monday.
No "I ruined everything."
Hydrate
Alcohol or salty foods dehydrate — water fixes this.
Weekends don't break consistency.
They strengthen your flexibility.

SECTION 4: HOW TO HANDLE VACATIONS
Vacations are where repaired metabolisms shine.
Eat breakfast EVERY day
Non-negotiable.
Keep protein in every meal
Even at restaurants.
Eat meals — don't graze all day
Grazing kills hunger signals.

Enjoy food guilt-free
You're supposed to LIVE.
Walk — a lot
Walking keeps digestion and hormones stable.
Drink more water
Heat, salt, travel all increase dehydration.
A healthy metabolism can handle:

- eating out
- different cuisines
- desserts
- irregular schedules

Why?
Because it's resilient.

SECTION 5: HOW TO HANDLE HOLIDAYS

Holidays are emotional, social, and food-heavy.
Here's the holiday guide:
Eat before the event
Don't show up starving.
Eat whole foods FIRST
Protein + carbs + veggies.
Dessert after.
No skipping meals
Skipping → bingeing.
Drink water throughout
Keeps hunger predictable.
Don't restrict the next day
Return to normal rhythm — NOT dieting.
One meal doesn't break you.
Returning to old patterns does.

SECTION 6: HOW TO HANDLE A "BAD DAY" OR SLIP

This is the biggest secret:

You don't start over.

You just return to consistency.

If you:

- overate
- binged
- skipped a meal
- had junk food
- ate at weird times
- went all day without enough protein
- stress-ate
- felt off

Here's the fix:

Next meal = whole food

Drink water

Return to rhythm

No guilt

No punishment

No starting over

No restrictions

You don't erase your progress unless you quit — and you're not quitting.

SECTION 7: WHEN TO TIGHTEN UP (AND WHEN NOT TO)

You tighten up when:

- hunger signals feel off
- cravings increase
- digestion becomes sluggish
- stress is unusually high

- sleep is poor
- meals become inconsistent
- you feel mentally scattered

Tightening up means:

- return to every 2–3 hour eating
- whole foods only
- increase water
- reduce fats temporarily
- increase carbs (fruit, rice, potatoes)
- lower intense exercise for 1–2 days

You DO NOT tighten up because:

- you had dessert
- you ate out
- you had a vacation
- you feel guilty
- you think you "should"
- you gained 1–3 pounds of water

A good metabolism is adaptive — NOT fragile.

SECTION 8: HOW TO KEEP YOUR RESULTS FOREVER

These are your lifelong anchors:

Anchor 1: Protein at every meal

Metabolic stability.

Anchor 2: Eat every 3–4 hours

Hormonal stability.

Anchor 3: Whole foods most of the time

Digestive stability.

Anchor 4: Walk daily

Cardiovascular + cortisol regulation.

Anchor 5: Sleep 7–9 hours

Hormonal repair.

Anchor 6: Hydration

Eliminates cravings, improves energy.

Anchor 7: No starving, no binging

Blood sugar control.

Anchor 8: Live your life

Flexibility protects mental health.

COACH'S CORNER

Look — you didn't come this far to go back to starving yourself.

You didn't come this far to return to dieting.

You didn't come this far to live scared of food again.

You healed your metabolism. You stabilized your hormones.

You broke the cycle that was breaking you.

Now live like it. Eat real food.

Eat consistently.

Fuel your body.

Trust your hunger.

And when life gets chaotic — come back to your rhythm.

This is your new life.

Not a diet.

Not a program.

Not a temporary fix.

A lifestyle you can live with forever.

Your metabolism is no longer your enemy — It's your power source.

Honor it.

Feed it.

Protect it.

Live with it.

You earned this.

FURTHER READING

Books, Articles, and Research for Deeper Understanding of Metabolism, Hormones, and Long-Term Weight Regulation

The following scientific and reader-friendly resources offer deeper insight into metabolism, hormonal regulation, nutrition, and sustainable weight loss. These works complement the principles of the Metabolism Reset and provide additional context from the fields of endocrinology, nutritional science, and behavioral psychology.

Scientific Articles & Journals

Adaptive Thermogenesis & Metabolic Adaptation

- Rosenbaum, M., & Leibel, R. L. (2010). Adaptive thermogenesis in humans. Obesity Reviews.
- Dulloo, A. G., & Jacquet, A. C. (1998). Adaptive reduction in basal metabolic rate in response to food deprivation. International Journal of Obesity.
- Fothergill, E., et al. (2016). Persistent metabolic adaptation 6 years after "The Biggest Loser" competition. Obesity.

Hunger Hormones & Appetite Regulation

- Klok, M. D., Jakobsdottir, S., & Drent, M. L. (2007). The role of leptin and ghrelin in the regulation of food intake and body weight. Journal of Clinical Endocrinology & Metabolism.
- Cummings, D. E., & Foster, K. E. (2003). Ghrelin and energy balance: The physiology of hunger. Nutrition Reviews.
- Friedman, J. (2014). Leptin and the regulation of body weight. American Journal of Clinical Nutrition.

Diet Failure & Weight Regain

- Mann, T., et al. (2007). Medicare's search for effective obesity treatments: Diets are not the answer. American Psychologist.
- Hall, K. D. (2016). Energy compensation and metabolic adaptation. American Journal of Clinical Nutrition.
- Polivy, J., & Herman, C. P. (multiple works on restraint theory).

Set Point Theory & Long-Term Regulation

- Sumithran, P., et al. (2011). Long-term persistence of hormonal adaptations to weight loss. New England Journal of Medicine.
- Speakman, J. R., & Levitsky, D. A. (2011). Set points, settling points, and the regulation of body weight. Obesity Reviews.

Books for General Readers
Metabolism & Nutrition
- Why We Get Fat — Gary Taubes
- Metabolical — Robert Lustig, MD
- Always Hungry? — David Ludwig, MD
- The Obesity Code — Jason Fung
- The Hungry Brain — Stephan Guyenet, PhD

Eating Behavior & Psychology
- Mindless Eating — Brian Wansink
- Intuitive Eating — Tribole & Resch
- Atomic Habits — James Clear
- The Willpower Instinct — Kelly McGonigal, PhD

Whole Foods & Nutrition Literacy
- Salt Sugar Fat — Michael Moss

- In Defense of Food — Michael Pollan
- The End of Overeating — David Kessler

Advanced Academic Reading
Metabolic Science

- Human Metabolism: A Regulatory Perspective — Keith N. Frayn
- Advanced Nutrition and Human Metabolism — Gropper & Smith

Exercise Physiology

- Exercise Metabolism — Brooks, Fahey, & Baldwin
- Essentials of Strength Training and Conditioning — NSCA

Behavioral Change & Sustainability

- Switch — Chip & Dan Heath
- Tiny Habits — BJ Fogg

Leonardo Lechuga

ACKNOWLEDGMENTS

I want to begin by acknowledging my family — my wife and my children. For most of my life, I have been driven by an almost unstoppable desire to build, provide, create, and conquer the world. And while that drive has taken me far, it has also meant that I wasn't always the husband or father they deserved. Yet through every chapter of my life, through every challenge and every reinvention, they never stopped believing in me. Their patience, love, and loyalty are the foundation under everything I've been able to accomplish. Thank you for standing with me while I learned, stumbled, grew, and kept pushing forward.

I want to acknowledge my upbringing and my parents. They were good people who did the best they could with the world they were handed. Growing up and watching them struggle lit a fire in me — not a fire of anger, but a fire of determination. I knew early on that I wanted more, not out of selfishness, but because I believed life had more to offer. That belief became the fuel that pushed me, clawed me forward, and shaped the man I would become.

I've also been blessed with mentors and people who believed in me long before I believed in myself. I want to thank Fred Morelli — the first person whose belief truly reached me. All my life, people told me I could do great things, but I never internalized those words until Fred spoke them. His confidence in me opened a door that changed everything. After him, I started letting encouragement in. I started believing that my future could be bigger than my past.

I want to thank David Blackburn for giving me my first real shot when I moved into a whole new environment. It was a different world, and he didn't just give me an opportunity — he

254

trusted me with it. That kind of belief becomes a turning point in a man's life.

And I want to acknowledge Jerry Moncus, who took me under his wing, supported my ambition, and encouraged my drive. He never tried to limit my thinking — he allowed me to be a free thinker, to build, to create, and to chase ideas bigger than myself. Every opportunity he opened for me became another step toward the life I'm living now.

To everyone who played a part, big or small, in shaping the man I am today — thank you. This book carries pieces of every lesson, every struggle, every victory, and every voice that pushed me forward. I am who I am because of all of you.

Leonardo Lechuga

www.ingramcontent.com/pod-product-compliance
Lightning Source LLC
Chambersburg PA
CBHW071307140726
47996CB00005B/1665